The ADHD Parenting Guide for Boys

© Copyright 2023 by Ginette Mendoza

Copyright © 2023 by Ginette Mendoza
All rights reserved. No part of this book may be reproduced, scanned,
or distributed in any printed or electronic form without permission.

First Edition: October 2023

Cover: Illustration made by Mike B.

Printed in the United States of America

TABLE OF CONTENTS

Dedicated to all my friends and to all the people
who gave me their help.
Thanks a lot
Thanks to all of you for your confidence
in my qualities and what I do.
Ginette Mendoza

CHAPTER 1

UNDERSTANDING ADHD IN BOYS

Defining ADHD: Symptoms, Types, and Diagnosis

Attention-Deficit Hyperactivity Disorder, commonly known as ADHD, is a neurodevelopmental disorder that predominantly begins in childhood and can continue into adulthood. This condition is characterized by persistent patterns of inattention, hyperactivity, and impulsivity that interfere with functioning or development.

ADHD is not a one-size-fits-all condition, it manifests differently in each individual. The symptoms can be categorized into two main groups: inattentive and hyperactive-impulsive. Inattentive symptoms include difficulty focusing, frequent mistakes, or forgetfulness, while hyperactive-impulsive symptoms can involve constant movement, interrupting others, and difficulty sitting still. However, it's important to understand that not all children with ADHD exhibit all these symptoms, and the severity can vary significantly.

The Diagnostic and Statistical Manual of Mental Disorders (DSM-5) identifies three types of ADHD: Predominantly Inattentive Presentation, Predominantly Hyperactive-Impulsive Presentation, and Combined Presentation.

The Predominantly Inattentive Presentation is characterized by symptoms such as difficulties with organization, sustaining attention, and following through on tasks. Children with this type of ADHD may seem to be daydreaming, forgetful, or careless.

In contrast, the Predominantly Hyperactive-Impulsive Presentation is marked by behaviors like fidgeting, talking excessively, and acting without consideration of consequences. These children might have trouble waiting their turn, frequently interrupt others, and struggle with sitting still.

The Combined Presentation, as the name suggests, is a mix of the inattentive and hyperactive-impulsive symptoms. Children with this type of ADHD display six or more symptoms from both categories.

Diagnosing ADHD is a multi-step process involving several types of evaluations, including medical examinations, interviews, behavior rating scales, and a thorough review of the child's developmental, social, and academic functioning. It's important to note that other conditions, like learning disabilities, anxiety, and depression, can coexist with ADHD or even mimic its symptoms, so a comprehensive assessment is vital for an accurate diagnosis.

In boys, ADHD can often manifest as disruptive behavior, making it more noticeable. Boys are more likely to be diagnosed with ADHD, not necessarily because they're more prone to the condition, but possibly because their symptoms are more overt. However, these behaviors can often be misinterpreted as willful disobedience or defiance, rather than symptoms of ADHD, leading to misunderstandings and missed opportunities for timely intervention and support.

It's crucial to debunk some common myths surrounding ADHD. It's not a result of bad parenting or lack of discipline, nor is it just about being hyperactive. ADHD is a legitimate neurodevelopmental disorder with a biological basis. It requires understanding, support, and often, professional intervention.

Parents and caregivers play a crucial role in the life of a child with ADHD. They can help their child cope with the challenges associated with the disorder by implementing structured routines, consistent rules, and positive reinforcement strategies. However, it's equally important for parents to take care of their own mental health, as dealing with ADHD can sometimes be overwhelming.

How ADHD Presents Differently in Boys

ADHD, or Attention Deficit Hyperactivity Disorder, is one of the most commonly diagnosed childhood psychiatric conditions. While ADHD occurs in both boys and girls, its presentation and symptoms often look different across genders. As a parent, it is crucial to understand how ADHD may uniquely impact your son.

Boys are two to three times more likely to be diagnosed with ADHD than girls. There are several reasons behind this disparity. Boys tend to exhibit more disruptive, externalizing behaviors associated with ADHD. They may be more hyperactive, impulsive, and inattentive in obvious, outward ways. Girls, on the other hand, are more likely to silently struggle with inattention. They frequently fly under the radar in classrooms, appearing spacey or ditzy rather than disruptive.

Additionally, expectations for boys' behavior in school environments tend to be stricter. Sitting still and concentrating for long periods goes against their energetic nature. Teachers are quicker to flag boys who cannot sit calmly compared to girls exhibiting similar restlessness. Diagnosis rates may also be higher for boys because parents and doctors look for ADHD more proactively in them.

Understanding how your son's ADHD symptoms may differ from a daughter's is key to getting him the right support. Here are some of the most common ways ADHD presents differently in boys.

Hyperactivity and Impulsivity

The hyperactive, impulsive symptoms of ADHD tend to be more overt in boys. As children, boys with ADHD often have trouble sitting still. You may notice your son constantly fidgeting, squirming in his seat, jumping up when he's meant to be seated, or running around at inappropriate times. Impulsivity can look like interrupting others frequently, shouting out answers before raising their hand, and generally poor emotional regulation.

Your son may also struggle with controlling his body and speech. He may talk excessively or make noises like humming without realizing it. Roughhousing, poking at classmates, and unfamiliarity with personal space are other common issues boys exhibit. Overall, these disruptive behaviors can hinder their learning and social interactions.

Inattention and Disorganization

While all children with ADHD struggle with inattention, boys again tend to display more external signs. Your son may have obvious difficulty sustaining focus in class or while doing homework. You'll notice his attention drifting within minutes, making it a battle to get through assignments.

Boys also tend to be more visibly disorganized than girls. Your son may regularly lose school supplies, forget to turn in homework, or struggle to keep his bedroom and belongings tidy. His backpack may become a black hole where important papers get lost. Following multi-step directions or completing tasks can be challenging for him.

These attention deficits and disorganization feed into each other, making school very difficult for boys with ADHD. Their assignments and notes may be messy or incomplete. Keeping track of due dates and schedules may be impossible without significant help.

Academic Difficulties

The visible symptoms of ADHD often directly translate into academic struggles for boys. Because hyperactivity, impulsivity, and inattention hinder learning, boys with ADHD are more likely to perform poorly and have difficulties in school.

Your son may have trouble mastering foundational academic skills, like reading, writing, and math. He may get distracted during lectures, forget information immediately, or struggle to understand instructions. Disorganization makes it harder to track assignments and meet deadlines. Careless errors may plague his work.

Frustration and low self-esteem may develop in classroom settings. Your son may act out to mask academic struggles. He requires more supervision, redirection, and individual support to succeed. Make sure to collaborate closely with his teachers and request adjustments where necessary.

Social Skill Deficits

Boys with ADHD often lag behind peers in social skills as well. Impulsivity can lead to inappropriate social behaviors, like interrupting conversations or being unable to wait their turn. Hyperactivity and trouble regulating emotions may make them seem immature. They may have trouble making or keeping friends.

Your son may also struggle picking up on social cues, unwritten rules, and subtleties in body language or tone. He may come across as inconsiderate or rude without meaning to. Friendly teasing or sarcasm tends to go over their heads. They have difficulty empathizing and putting themselves in others' shoes.

Work on explaining social rules clearly to your son. Role play appropriate interactions with him. Provide constructive feedback when he makes social faux pas. Building these skills will help him connect better with peers.

Excitability and Emotional Dysregulation

Boys with ADHD tend to be more excitable and quick to react emotionally. Your son may get silly and wound up in environments with too much stimulation. When over-excited, he may have trouble calming himself down.

Emotional outbursts, both positive and negative, may seem extreme. Your son may shout, cry, or even tantrum when frustrated. Anger, disappointment, worry, and other difficult feelings may overwhelm him. Coping strategies for managing emotions will be important to teach.

On the positive end, your son may be exuberant when excited. Holidays or special events can become chaotic without measured expectations set. Always brace for excitement and emotionally intensified reactions.

Sleep Issues

Sleep troubles are common with ADHD, but tend to affect boys more prominently. Your son may have difficulty settling down at night due to constant motion and stimulation-seeking. Hyperactivity persists around bedtime. Even when exhausted, boys struggle to relax.

Once asleep, boys with ADHD tend to be restless sleepers. They switch positions frequently. Bed-wetting, talking in their sleep, or waking up often throughout the night can also occur. Sleep quality suffers, leading to daytime drowsiness.

Establishing calming bedtime routines is essential. Limit screen time before bed, encourage reading, and set consistent sleep and wake times. If sleep issues persist, speak to your pediatrician. Getting good rest is crucial for managing ADHD.

Difference in Disease Severity

Studies suggest that boys not only show more outward signs of ADHD, their symptoms also tend to be more severe in nature overall. Boys exhibit greater problems with inattention and hyperactivity that distinctly impact life functioning. The part of the brain impacted by ADHD tends to differ in size between boys and girls.

However, it is important to remember that ADHD presents as a spectrum in both genders. Your son may have mild, moderate, or severe ADHD requiring different levels of support. Do not assume every boy with ADHD fits one universal mold. There is significant individual variation within the diagnosis.

Increased Risk of Co-Occurring Disorders

The externalizing behaviors of ADHD in boys tend to increase their risk of developing certain co-occurring conditions as well:

- Learning disabilities like dyslexia are more common in boys with ADHD. Challenges with reading, writing, math, or other subjects may require special academic support.

- Symptoms of autism spectrum disorder and ADHD frequently overlap in boys. Social and communication difficulties may accompany ADHD.

- Oppositional defiant disorder involves extreme stubbornness, anger, resentfulness, and arguing with authority figures. It occurs more frequently in boys with ADHD.

- Conduct disorder features more extreme rule-breaking and antisocial behaviors like aggression or destruction of property. It is strongly associated with ADHD in boys.

If you notice other pronounced struggles beyond classic ADHD symptoms, consult a psychologist about possible co-morbid diagnoses. Catching these early allows for proper treatment.

The Middle School Cliff

As boys with ADHD progress through late elementary school, major challenges often arise around middle school. The transition to switching classrooms with different teachers is extremely difficult. The volume of work and organizational skills required ramps up significantly. Independence is expected, but hard to achieve with executive functioning deficits.

Because of these factors, ADHD symptoms often worsen around sixth grade for boys. Make sure to provide extra support and advocacy during this rocky transition. Work closely with the school to put accommodations in place. oregano Some tutoring or therapy may also help overcome this cliff.

Puberty and Hormones

The onset of puberty brings major biological and emotional changes for all boys, with or without ADHD. But for boys with ADHD, the effects of surging hormones tend to exacerbate their symptoms.

As testosterone increases through puberty, you may notice your son's impulsivity, aggression, and defiance worsening for a time. Challenging behaviors likely increase as he adjusts to the new feelings and pressures of adolescence. His organizational skills may temporarily decline further.

While frustrating to manage, understand that this increase in symptoms is a normal phase rather than regression. Provide him extra patience and guidance during puberty, and consult his doctor if the changes become unmanageable. Once his hormones balance out, he will likely return to his baseline ADHD symptom levels.

The Impact of ADHD on a Child's Life

For children diagnosed with ADHD, their everyday reality is often fraught with challenges that can touch every aspect of their lives. This chapter aims to provide a comprehensive overview of the ways ADHD can influence a child's social, academic, and emotional world, while offering practical advice to help navigate these impacts.

ADHD is not merely a condition that affects a child's ability to pay attention or sit still. It's a complex disorder that can significantly impact a child's life in various ways. Let's delve into some of these impacts to better understand the challenges a child with ADHD might face.

Academic Challenges

Academic challenges are often one of the most noticeable impacts of ADHD. Difficulties with focus and attention can make it hard for a child to keep up with schoolwork, follow instructions, and complete tasks. They may often overlook details in their work, leading to frequent mistakes. Organizational skills can also be a challenge, making it hard to keep track of assignments and materials. Homework can become a battleground, with procrastination and avoidance becoming common issues.

Social Challenges

ADHD can also affect a child's social interactions. Impulsivity may lead to interrupting others, not waiting for their turn, or acting without considering the consequences. This behavior can make it difficult for them to make and keep friends. They may also struggle to pick up on social cues, leading to misunderstandings and conflicts.

Emotional Challenges

Children with ADHD often experience emotional dysregulation, which means they have difficulty managing their emotions. They may have intense emotional reactions to situations, experience frequent mood swings, or have trouble calming down after an upset. This emotional volatility can be confusing and distressing for the child and those around them.

Self-Esteem Issues

The constant struggle with academics, social interactions, and emotions can lead to feelings of frustration, failure, and low self-esteem in children with ADHD. They may start to view themselves as different or less capable than their peers, which can further exacerbate their challenges.

Despite these challenges, it's important to remember that ADHD does not define a child. They have their unique strengths and capabilities. The key is to foster these strengths while providing support and strategies to manage the challenges. Here are some practical ways to do this:

Academic Support

Work closely with your child's teachers to understand the challenges your child is facing at school. Implementing an Individualized Education Plan (IEP) or a 504 plan can provide accommodations to help your child succeed academically. At home, establish a quiet and clutter-free homework area, use visual aids for task management, and break assignments into manageable parts.

Social Skills Training

Help your child develop social skills by role-playing different scenarios, discussing appropriate responses, and providing feedback. Encourage participation in structured activities where they can interact with peers under supervision.

Emotional Regulation Strategies

Teach your child techniques for managing emotions, such as deep breathing, mindfulness, and other self-calming strategies. Provide a safe and non-judgemental space for them to express their feelings.

Boosting Self-Esteem

Focus on your child's strengths and celebrate their successes, no matter how small. Encourage hobbies and activities where they can shine. Constantly remind them that everyone has their own strengths and weaknesses, and having ADHD is just one part of who they are.

Living with ADHD presents unique challenges for a child. But with understanding, support, and the right strategies, these challenges can be managed. It's important for parents, teachers, and caregivers to remember that every child with ADHD has the potential to grow into a successful and fulfilled adult. Their journey might be a bit different – but it's a journey that can be filled with achievements, growth, and joy.

ADHD and Co-Occurring Conditions

ADHD rarely travels alone. It often comes with one or more co-occurring conditions, making the understanding and management of ADHD more complex. This chapter sheds light on some common conditions that often coexist with ADHD, and provides practical strategies to address them.

Learning Disabilities

Learning disabilities, such as dyslexia, dysgraphia, and dyscalculia, are often found in individuals with ADHD. These disabilities can make it difficult for a child to read, write, or perform mathematical calculations, respectively. These challenges can further amplify the academic difficulties experienced by a child with ADHD.

Anxiety Disorders

Anxiety disorders are another common co-occurring condition with ADHD. Children with ADHD and anxiety may feel excessively worried or fearful. This anxiety can interfere with their daily activities. Moreover, their ADHD symptoms, such as forgetfulness or difficulties in school, can further fuel their anxiety.

Depression

Children with ADHD are also at a higher risk of experiencing depression. The constant struggle with ADHD symptoms and the resulting difficulties can lead to feelings of sadness, hopelessness, or a lack of interest in activities they once enjoyed.

Oppositional Defiant Disorder (ODD)

Some children with ADHD may also have Oppositional Defiant Disorder. Children with ODD show a pattern of defiant, hostile, and disobedient behavior toward authority figures. This can lead to frequent conflicts at home and school.

Autism Spectrum Disorder (ASD)

While less common, Autism Spectrum Disorder can co-occur with ADHD. ASD is a developmental disorder that affects communication and behavior. Children with both ADHD and ASD may face additional challenges in social interaction, communication, and repetitive behaviors.

Understanding these co-occurring conditions is crucial because they can influence the severity of ADHD symptoms and the effectiveness of treatment strategies. Therefore, a comprehensive evaluation that considers potential co-occurring conditions is essential for an accurate diagnosis and treatment plan. Here are some strategies to manage these conditions:

Early Intervention

Early intervention is key. If you suspect your child has a co-occurring condition, seek professional help right away. Early diagnosis and treatment can make a significant difference in your child's development and quality of life.

Integrated Treatment Approach

An integrated treatment approach addresses both ADHD and the co-occurring condition. This approach can involve medication, behavioral therapy, educational support, and self-care strategies.

Consistent Routine

A consistent routine can provide a sense of security and predictability for a child with ADHD and co-occurring conditions. This routine can include regular times for meals, homework, play, and sleep.

Social and Emotional Support

Provide ample social and emotional support. Encourage your child to express their feelings and reassure them that it's okay to feel upset or anxious. Teach them coping strategies and problem-solving skills.

Collaboration with Professionals

Collaborate with professionals such as teachers, therapists, and doctors. They can provide valuable insights and guidance to manage your child's ADHD and co-occurring conditions.

It's worth noting that while these co-occurring conditions add another layer of complexity to ADHD, they can also provide a broader understanding of a child's behavior and needs. This understanding can open doors to tailored strategies and interventions that address the unique challenges faced by a child with ADHD and co-occurring conditions.

ADHD, Boys, and the Education System

Navigating school is challenging for any child, but for boys with ADHD, the traditional education system often exacerbates their struggles. The long hours sitting still, organizational demands, noise and stimulation, and social dynamics are not designed with their needs in mind. As a parent, being your son's advocate within this complex system is essential.

Know that with the right support, accommodation, and strategies, your boy can absolutely thrive academically and socially in school. It simply takes proper understanding of his needs, open communication with staff, and creativity in adapting the environment to allow his neurodiverse mind to shine.

Common Classroom Challenges for Boys with ADHD

- **Sitting still:** The expectation to remain seated for hours goes against boys' energetic nature. Desks and chairs can feel like torture devices to them.

- **Focusing:** Their attention drifts within minutes, even during activities they enjoy. Constant re-focusing is exhausting.

- **Organization:** Keeping track of materials, assignments, and due dates is enormously difficult. Their work and backpacks become disorganized chaos.

- **Distractions:** Noisy classmates, sights, smells, or thoughts can constantly pull their attention from the task at hand. Filtering stimuli is hard.

- **Transitions:** Switching between activities or classes is hugely challenging. They cannot shift mindsets quickly.

- **Social cues:** Reading body language, social subtleties, and unspoken rules often confuses them. Social dynamics are an enigma.

- **Self-control:** Impulsiveness and emotional regulation are limited. Outbursts or inappropriate behaviors happen without thinking.

- **Memory:** Retaining and recalling information from short-term memory is compromised. Instructions, facts, and details slip away quickly.

- **Discouragement:** Criticism, punishment, and frustrations around failure can take a huge toll on self-esteem. School often damages, not builds, confidence.

Seeking Accommodations

By law, your son's public school must provide "reasonable accommodations" through a 504 Plan or IEP to help him succeed academically. Don't be afraid to assertively request adjustments like:

- Frequent breaks to move around

- Alternative seating options (exercise ball, standing desk)

- Reduced assignments and modified tests

- Additional time for assignments and testing

- Teacher notes, study guides, or copies of slides provided

- Visual supports like behavior charts

- Supervised organizational help

- Quiet study space to take tests

- Noise-cancelling headphones to reduce distraction

Your child has a right to the accommodations that will allow him to perform at grade level. Always approach teachers from a standpoint of collaborative problem-solving. Make sure to acknowledge their efforts and demands as well.

Executive Functioning Strategies

Boys with ADHD often struggle with executive functioning skills like organization, time management, planning, and working memory. Build these skills explicitly:

- Use planners religiously. Break assignments into steps over time. Set reminders for everything.

- Clean out backpacks every night and reorganize. Have a folder/binder for each subject.

- Allow extra time for transitions. Alert him 5-10 minutes before switching tasks.

- Give one-step instructions. Have him repeat back directions. Provide visual or written prompts.

- Help him build habits. Consistent routines are key. Post checklists and reminders everywhere.

- Reduce clutter at home and in the classroom. Visual overload distracts.

- Celebrate effort and progress. Don't criticize - it corrodes self-esteem.

Physical Activity and Learning

Physical activity powerfully enhances cognitive function and learning in boys with ADHD. Find regular opportunities during the school day to get them moving:

- Schedule outdoor recess as often as possible, at least 20-30 minutes per day.

- Incorporate brain breaks between lessons with exercises or games. Even 5 minutes is beneficial.

- Allow movement during class through standing desks, exercise balls, or the ability to pace while working.

- Build physical education, intramural sports, or recess time into after-school care schedules.

- Teach them mindful breathing techniques to use anytime as "body breaks."

Studies consistently show improved focus, memory, and hyperactivity control when physical activity is interwoven with academics. Movement opens pathways for learning.

Managing Stimulus and Distraction

The traditional classroom offers sensory overload for ADHD brains. Work with teachers to manage stimulation:

- Allow the use of noise-cancelling headphones to reduce auditory distractions.

- Permit doodling or fidget toys during lessons to channel excess energy.

- Simplify visual environments by reducing wall displays.

- Provide preferential seating away from doors, windows, or talkative peers.

- Offer quiet study corners or tents within the classroom.

- Use room dividers, study carrels, or partitions to create defined workspaces.

- Permit standing desks in the back to allow movement without disrupting others.

Customizing the environment reduces overload and enables better focus. Allowing tactile/auditory outlets like doodling or music also helps concentration immensely.

Positive Behavior Reinforcement

Boys with ADHD respond extremely well to positive reinforcement systems. Traditional punitive discipline backfires by worsening behaviors and self-image. Work with teachers to implement:

- A token economy system. Boys earn rewards (stickers, points, coins) for positive behaviors which translate into prizes.

- Clear expectations paired with regular praise for effort. Boys should know exactly what merits acknowledgement.

- Private visual behavior charts at their desk tracking goals and progress. Review and reset goals together.

- Home/school communication logs to give parents opportunities to reinforce school behaviors at home.

- Celebrations for achievement like Student of the Week awards or certificates to recognize progress.

With a supportive system highlighting effort and improvement, boys can develop confidence and skills for success.

Prioritizing Social-Emotional Learning

Academic skill building is only one piece of the puzzle. Ensure teachers also prioritize emotional awareness, friendship skills, self-esteem building, and coping strategies explicitly through:

- Social skills groups to practice strategies like conversation or sharing.

- Role playing positive interactions and problem-solving conflict.

- Journaling, art therapy, or discussion groups to explore feelings.

- Confidence-building lessons focused on identifying strengths.

- Relaxation and mindfulness practices during class.

- Emotional check-ins during the day.

Developing social-emotional intelligence helps boys feel connected, understood, and valued. A sense of belonging is critical.

As a parent, you are the lynchpin making school work for an ADHD child. Arm yourself with knowledge of effective strategies. Build rapport with teachers. Communicate concerns quickly. You have the power to shape an environment where your unique, amazing son will succeed on all fronts.

Debunking Common ADHD Myths

ADHD, despite being a well-studied medical condition, is surrounded by a myriad of misconceptions. These myths can perpetuate stigma, lead to misdiagnosis, and hinder effective treatment. This chapter aims to debunk some common ADHD myths and shed light on the realities behind them.

Myth 1: ADHD Isn't a Real Disorder

ADHD is indeed a real and recognized medical condition. It's a neurodevelopmental disorder characterized by symptoms of inattention, impulsivity, and hyperactivity. The American Psychiatric Association, World Health Organization, and other medical organizations recognize it as a legitimate diagnosis. Brain imaging studies have even shown structural and functional differences in the brains of individuals with ADHD.

Myth 2: Only Hyperactive Boys Have ADHD

While ADHD is often diagnosed in boys during their early school years, it's not exclusive to them. Girls can have ADHD too, but their symptoms might present differently, often leading to underdiagnosis. Also, not all individuals with ADHD exhibit hyperactivity. There are three types of ADHD: predominantly inattentive, predominantly hyperactive/impulsive, and combined type.

Myth 3: People with ADHD Just Need to Try Harder

ADHD is not a result of laziness or lack of motivation. It's a neurobiological condition that affects a person's executive functions, making it difficult to plan, focus, and control impulses. Telling someone with ADHD to "try harder" is like telling someone with poor eyesight to squint harder to see clearly. They need appropriate interventions and support, not just effort.

Myth 4: Children Outgrow ADHD

While symptoms of ADHD can change over time, many individuals continue to experience them into adulthood. Approximately two-thirds of children with ADHD continue to grapple with the disorder in their adult years. These adults might struggle with time management, organization, self-control, and other areas impacted by ADHD.

Myth 5: Medication is the Only Treatment for ADHD

Medication can be a crucial part of managing ADHD, but it's not the only treatment option. Behavioral interventions, lifestyle changes, counseling, and educational support can also be effective. In many cases, a multi-modal approach that combines several strategies is recommended.

Understanding these myths is the first step towards debunking them. It's essential to educate ourselves and others about the realities of ADHD to promote empathy, understanding, and effective support for those living with this condition. Here are some ways to do this:

Educate Yourself and Others

Learn about ADHD from reliable sources, such as scientific journals, reputable health websites, and healthcare professionals. Share this knowledge with others to help dispel myths.

Advocate for ADHD Awareness

Promote ADHD awareness in your community, school, or workplace. This could involve organizing informational sessions, sharing resources, or supporting ADHD-friendly policies.

Support Individuals with ADHD

Offer support to individuals with ADHD. This could include understanding their challenges, offering help when needed, and treating them with kindness and respect.

Seek Professional Guidance

If you or someone you know has ADHD, seek guidance from healthcare professionals. They can provide accurate information, diagnose the condition, and offer treatment options.

CHAPTER 2

THE EMOTIONAL WORLD OF BOYS WITH ADHD

ADHD and Emotional Dysregulation

ADHD is often associated with inattention, hyperactivity, and impulsivity. However, another critical aspect of ADHD that is sometimes overlooked is emotional dysregulation. Emotional dysregulation refers to difficulties in managing emotional responses. For those with ADHD, these difficulties can result in emotional responses that are more intense, last longer, and are less appropriate to the situation than those of their peers.

Understanding Emotional Dysregulation in ADHD

Emotional dysregulation can manifest in various ways, such as intense emotional reactions, difficulty calming down after an upset, or problems transitioning from one emotion to another. Individuals with ADHD may also have a lower frustration tolerance, leading to outbursts or meltdowns over seemingly minor issues.

Impact of Emotional Dysregulation

The impacts of emotional dysregulation can be far-reaching. It can affect relationships, academic performance, self-esteem, and mental health. For example, a child who has frequent emotional outbursts may struggle to make friends, leading to feelings of loneliness and low self-esteem. In the long term, these issues can contribute to the development of secondary conditions, such as anxiety or depression.

Causes of Emotional Dysregulation in ADHD

The exact cause of emotional dysregulation in ADHD is not fully understood. However, it's believed to be related to differences in brain structure and function. Specifically, the areas of the brain responsible for emotional regulation may be less active or smaller in individuals with ADHD.

Despite the challenges posed by emotional dysregulation, there are strategies that can help individuals with ADHD manage their emotions more effectively. These include:

Cognitive Behavioral Therapy (CBT)

CBT is a type of psychotherapy that can help individuals with ADHD recognize their patterns of thinking and how these patterns influence their emotions and behavior. By changing unhelpful thought patterns, they can learn to respond to situations in a more adaptive way.

Mindfulness Practices

Mindfulness involves paying attention to the present moment without judgment. Mindfulness practices, such as meditation or deep breathing exercises, can help individuals with ADHD manage their emotions by promoting relaxation and increasing self-awareness.

Social Skills Training

Social skills training can help individuals with ADHD learn appropriate emotional responses. This training typically involves role-playing scenarios and practicing emotional responses.

Medication

In some cases, medication may be an effective adjunct to behavioral strategies in managing emotional dysregulation in ADHD. However, this decision should be made in consultation with a healthcare professional.

Self-Care

Self-care practices, such as getting regular exercise, maintaining a healthy diet, and ensuring adequate sleep, can also help manage emotional dysregulation. These practices can improve overall mood and enhance the body's ability to cope with stress.

Living with emotional dysregulation can be challenging, but with the right support and strategies, individuals with ADHD can learn to manage their emotions effectively. It's essential to approach emotional dysregulation with understanding and compassion, recognizing that it's a legitimate and challenging aspect of ADHD.

Understanding Your Child's Feelings

Understanding a child's feelings is crucial to their emotional development and the building of a strong parent-child bond. Children, especially younger ones, may not yet have the vocabulary or understanding to express their feelings adequately. Therefore, it's up to the adults in their life to help them navigate their emotions and teach them how to express themselves in healthy, constructive ways.

The Importance of Understanding Your Child's Feelings

Developing emotional intelligence in your child is as vital as teaching them to read and write. It aids in their social interactions, builds their self-esteem, and equips them with the necessary tools to handle life's challenges. By understanding your child's feelings, you can guide them in recognizing, expressing, and managing their emotions appropriately.

Steps to Understand Your Child's Feelings

- **Observe Their Behavior:** Children often express their feelings through behavior. A sudden change in behavior, such as increased aggression or withdrawal, may indicate that your child is grappling with complex emotions.

- **Listen Actively:** When your child talks about their feelings, listen attentively and show that you're interested. This will encourage them to express themselves more openly and honestly.

- **Validate Their Feelings:** Even if a child's feelings seem irrational to you, they are real to them. By validating their feelings, you show them that it's okay to have emotions and to express them.

- **Help Them Label Their Feelings:** Young children might not have the words to express their feelings. Help them by naming the emotion you think they're experiencing.

- **Teach Them Emotional Regulation:** Once your child can identify their emotions, teach them healthy ways to manage these feelings. This could involve deep breathing, taking a break, or talking about their feelings.

The Challenges of Understanding a Child's Feelings

Understanding a child's feelings can sometimes be challenging, particularly when their feelings seem disproportionate to the situation or when they have trouble expressing themselves. During these times, it's important to remain patient and empathetic. Remember that emotional development is a process, and each child will mature at their own pace.

How to Navigate Difficult Emotions

Some feelings, such as sadness, anger, or fear, can be particularly difficult for a child to handle. In these instances, it's crucial to provide comfort and reassurance while guiding them towards understanding and managing these emotions. This can be a teaching moment where you demonstrate that everyone experiences such emotions and it's perfectly okay.

The Role of Play in Understanding Emotions

Play provides a safe space for children to express and work through their feelings. Encourage imaginative play where they can role-play different scenarios. This will not only help them express their feelings but also develop empathy by understanding others' emotions.

Fostering Emotional Intelligence

Emotional dysregulation is a common challenge for children with ADHD. The condition makes it difficult to identify, process, and modulate feelings appropriately. For boys, intense emotions may spiral into verbal or physical outbursts without the ability to self-regulate. Teaching your son emotional intelligence skills allows him to understand his inner world better while avoiding meltdowns.

What Does Emotional Intelligence Involve?

Emotional intelligence is the ability to:

- Identify and label feelings in yourself and others.

- Express emotions constructively through words or actions.

- Regulate impulses and behave appropriately despite difficult feelings.

- Empathize with others and show compassion.

- Persevere through setbacks using coping strategies.

Mastering these competencies leads to greater self-awareness, resiliency, healthy relationships, and success in all areas of life.

Why Emotional Intelligence Matters

For boys with ADHD, building emotional intelligence should be a top priority in their development. Struggles with emotional control and impulsiveness lead to:

- Difficulty maintaining friendships.

- Acting out behaviors and temper tantrums.

- Disciplinary issues at home and school.

- Low self-confidence and negative mindsets.

- Family conflicts and damaged relationships.

Emotional competency gives boys the tools to process feelings in constructive ways instead. They become better equipped to handle life's ups and downs.

Teaching Emotion Identification

Many boys struggle simply identifying emotions within themselves or others. Start by building a feelings vocabulary using:

- Flashcards with feeling faces. Name the emotions together.

- Stories and books exploring feelings. Stop to discuss how characters feel.

- Mirroring faces showing different emotions and having him guess which one.

- Music and art therapy to identify moods.

Also encourage noticing physical cues, like body sensations, associated with feelings. Help him connect emotions with the situations that trigger them. Over time, consciousfeeling identification will come more naturally to him.

Encouraging Emotional Expression

Boys often mask or bottle up their feelings. Give your son healthy outlets for expression by:

- Validating all emotions as normal and human. Never shame.

- Practicing "I feel..." sentence stems to discuss emotions.

- Modeling talking about your own feelings calmly.

- Writing, drawing, or storytelling to express emotions indirectly if needed.

- Role playing healthy expression through body language and tone.

Letting him authentically articulate feelings prevents internalizing or acting out. Create an open, non-judgmental space for processing emotions.

Teaching Self-Regulation Strategies

When emotions intensify, the ability to self-soothe allows boys to cope and re-center. Strategies include:

- Taking deep breaths. Have him slowly inhale through his nose and exhale through his mouth.

- Going for a walk or run. Physical activity naturally calms the nervous system.

- Listening to soothing music.

- Hugging a stuffed animal or blanket.

- Talking to himself in an encouraging tone.

- Calling a trusted friend or family member.

- Using a stress ball or fidget toy.

Build a "coping skills toolbox" he can access anytime emotions spike. The ability to self-regulate will prevent many behaviour issues.

Role-Playing Challenging Situations

Rehearse handling difficult social and emotional scenarios through practice. Common examples include:

- Dealing with disappointment when something desired is denied.

- Coping when friends cannot play or plans get cancelled.

- Accepting imperfection, like making a mistake on schoolwork.

- Experiencing peer conflict and navigating resolution respectfully.

- Receiving constructive criticism or negative feedback.

Practice self-talk, breathing, and healthy responses. Talk through alternative reactions. Facing simulations in role plays builds skills for real-world application.

Encouraging Empathy

The ability to empathize allows boys to understand others' realities. Build empathy through:

- Discussing characters' perspectives in books and movies.

- Considering how words or actions affect others before reacting.

- Role reversal scenarios exploring how he would feel.

- Putting himself in someone else's shoes visually by sketching or writing.

- Volunteering to help those in need, like at a food bank.

Use discipline as an opportunity to build empathy by reflecting on how his actions impacted others. Linking emotions to outcomes teaches compassion.

Managing Anger and Frustration

For boys with ADHD, anger or annoyance often manifest physically through yelling, aggression, or destructive behavior. Strategies for dealing with frustration include:

- Taking a break from the situation to calm down.

- Squeezing a stress ball or pillow.

- Running laps or doing push ups.

-Listening to music.

- Drawing or writing about the anger.

- Talking it through with you after cooling off.

- Apologizing to anyone affected once emotions have settled.

Equip your son with healthy mechanisms for channeling anger productively. Removing himself from the situation prevents reactive escalations.

Fostering Positive Self-Talk

Boys with ADHD often battle negative self-perception and criticism. Teach self-affirming self-talk to cultivate emotional resilience. Examples include:

- "I am strong and capable."

- "Mistakes help me learn."

- "I can handle this challenge."

- "My effort matters more than results."

- "It's okay to feel this way. My feelings are normal."

- "I can always try again."

Post reminders with positive phrases everywhere - his bedroom, the fridge, backpack. Counter the inner critic with empowering messages.

Modeling Emotional Intelligence

As a parent, your boy will mimic your emotional responses. Strive to continually model:

- Staying calm during conflict.

- Talking through anger instead of yelling.

- Admitting when you make mistakes.

- Being kind, respectful, and forgiving to yourself and others.

- Apologizing for overreactions.

- Taking care of yourself when stressed.

Your example shapes his development profoundly. Show him how fulfilling life is when living with emotional intelligence.

Though emotional regulation presents challenges for boys with ADHD, skill building lays the groundwork for mastering their inner world. Have patience on the journey. With your guidance, empathy, and support, your son can learn to harness his emotions as a superpower, not a weakness.

Coping with Anger and Frustration

In the journey of life, anger and frustration are inevitable emotions that everyone encounters. They may arise from various circumstances, including unmet expectations, feeling unheard or disrespected, or simply having a bad day. While these emotions are normal and part of the human experience, managing them effectively is crucial for maintaining mental health and fostering healthy relationships.

Understanding Anger and Frustration

Anger is a strong emotion that is often a response to a perceived threat or injustice. Frustration, on the other hand, typically arises from feeling blocked or impeded in some way. Both of these emotions can lead to discomfort and, if not managed wisely, can result in negative consequences, such as damaged relationships, health issues, or even legal problems.

The Impact of Anger and Frustration

Beyond the immediate effects, chronic anger and frustration can have long-term implications. These emotions can lead to stress, anxiety, depression, and physical health issues such as heart disease. They can also negatively impact relationships, both personally and professionally, leading to isolation and loneliness.

Self-Awareness: The First Step in Managing Anger and Frustration

Recognizing and acknowledging your anger and frustration is the first step in managing these emotions. Pay attention to the physical signs such as increased heart rate, clenched fists, or feeling hot. Also, notice the thoughts and situations that trigger these emotions in you.

Techniques to Cope with Anger and Frustration

- **Deep Breathing:** When you notice the signs of anger and frustration, take a few moments to breathe deeply. This can help to calm your body and mind, giving you a chance to respond rather than react.

- **Mindfulness:** Mindfulness involves being fully present in the moment, without judgment. This can help you to observe your emotions objectively and to let them pass without acting on them.

- **Physical Activity:** Regular exercise can help to reduce feelings of anger and frustration by releasing tension and boosting your mood.

- **Cognitive Restructuring:** This involves changing the way you think about the situation that is causing your anger or frustration. Instead of focusing on the negative, try to find a more positive or neutral perspective.

- **Problem Solving:** If your anger or frustration is caused by a specific problem, try to find a solution. This might involve seeking advice, making a plan, or taking action.

Professional Help for Managing Anger and Frustration

Sometimes, despite your best efforts, anger and frustration may continue to be a significant issue. In such cases, it may be helpful to seek professional help. Therapists and counselors can provide strategies and tools to manage these emotions effectively.

Building a Positive Self-Image

Boys with ADHD often struggle with low self-esteem and negative self-talk. The challenges of ADHD - school struggles, social difficulties, emotional outbursts - can corrode confidence over time. As a parent, building your son's positive self-image is critical to help him know his worth. Though ADHD brings certain weaknesses, redirect focus onto appreciating strengths, talents, and uniqueness.

The Roots of Negative Self-Image

Multiple factors commonly damage self-perception in boys with ADHD:

- Criticism and correction from authority figures like teachers or coaches.

- Feeling different from peers or left out of social activities.

- Poor academic performance leading to shame or discouragement.

- Impulsiveness resulting in frequent disciplining.

- Hyperfocusing on mistakes and flaws due to perfectionism.

- Listening to the inner critic's persistent negativity.

Over time, these influencers breed an attitude of self-blame, poor self-worth, and identity confusion. Your son needs you to counteract these voices.

Signs of Negative Self-Perception

Watch for both emotional and behavioral indicators of low self-esteem:

- Expressing self-criticism frequently through negative self-talk.

- Excessive reluctance to try new things for fear of failure.

- Withdrawing from social situations due to embarrassment.

- Perfectionistic over-focus on errors or flaws in performance.

- Extreme sensitivity to criticism or negative feedback.

- Changes in eating habits, sleep, or mental health.

- Acting out behaviors to gain acceptance or control.

The sooner you notice symptoms emerging, the quicker you can intervene with positivity.

Accepting the ADHD Diagnosis

A pivotal first step is encouraging your son to embrace his neurodiversity as a difference, not a disadvantage. Frame ADHD in a strengths-based way:

- His brain is wired to be creative, energetic, and passionate.

- ADHD gives him unique gifts and talents.

- With the right environment and tools, he can thrive with ADHD.

- Use role models with ADHD who found success.

Make sure he knows his diagnosis does not define or limit him. Forging a positive ADHD identity builds self-worth.

Celebrating Strengths and Talents

Help your son recognize abilities and personal qualities he excels in:

- Creative talents like art, writing, music, or crafting.

- Athletic prowess in sports, dance, or physical activities.

- Interpersonal strengths like humor, enthusiasm, or friendliness.

- Advanced intellectual skills such as problem-solving, strategy, or spatial skills.

Build his confidence by encouraging activities he enjoys and shines at. Passion fuels positivity. Provide opportunities to showcase strengths among supportive people.

Shifting Focus from Weaknesses

Boys with ADHD fixate on where they fall short. Guide your son to redirect thoughts from weaknesses to strengths through:

- Making lists of positive qualities, talents, and skills to revisit.

- Tracking accomplishments in a confidence journal. Re-read when needing a boost.

- Writing encouraging notes on mirrors or walls to see daily.

- Putting energy into building strengths rather than obsessing over deficits.

- Surrounding himself with friends and mentors who see his strengths.

The mental habit of highlighting abilities takes practice but prevents negativity spirals.

Cultivating Positive Self-Talk

The constant inner critic is a core driver of poor self-image. Boys believe these exaggerated negative messages. Arm your son against destructive self-talk by:

- Teaching him to identify maladaptive thoughts and verbalize more accurate statements.

- Practicing reframing negative self-talk in the moment. Write empowering alternatives on cards to reference.

- Making lists of positive affirmations. Have him repeat them daily.

- Using positive visualization to imagine achieving goals.

- Writing letters of encouragement to himself to re-read when needed.

Repetitive positive messages will transform his inner monologue over time.

Seeking Healthy Validation

All boys need regular doses of external validation to fuel their self-concept. Provide consistent praise and encouragement around:

- Effort, perseverance, and hard work. These build confidence.

- Meeting responsibilities or goals, however small. Progress fuels motivation.

- Acts of kindness, patience, integrity, or other values. Character matters.

- Showing emotional maturity and regulation during difficult moments.

Let praise significantly outweigh criticism. Emphasize that his value is not dependent on achievement or perfection.

Becoming the Positive Voice

The most powerful way to nurture self-esteem is by becoming the dominant positive voice in your son's mind. Provide a continuous stream of:

- Praise and appreciation for his uniqueness.

- Unconditional love and belief in his abilities.

- Support picking him up after setbacks or failures.

- Focus on strengths and potential during challenges.

- Pride in the person he is becoming.

With you actively countering the inner critic, his self-perception will flourish.

Modeling Self-Confidence and Self-Care

Your relationship with yourself serves as your son's template for self-image. Model:

- Speaking positively about your body.

- Celebrating your strengths and accomplishments.

- Exuding self-assurance in your worth and abilities.

- Not beating yourself up over mistakes.

- Setting boundaries against criticism or toxicity.

- Making self-care a priority every day.

- Surrounding yourself with people who appreciate you.

Your words and actions teach him how to build his own self-esteem.

Seeking Professional Help When Needed

If low self-worth leads to depression, anxiety, self-harm, or other sustained issues impacting health and relationships, seek counseling. Therapists can provide tools to help transform harmful thought patterns. There is no shame in needing extra support.

Remember, your son's self-concept is malleable. With consistent nurturing, he can bloom into a young man grounded in his self-worth. Cultivate an environment where his strengths and talents are spotlighted and celebrated. The seeds you plant today will blossom into an unshakeable sense of identity and pride. Keep watering them with positivity.

CHAPTER 3

NAVIGATING THE EDUCATIONAL LANDSCAPE

Challenges Faced in Traditional Learning Environments

Traditional learning environments, where teaching is often one-sided with instructors imparting knowledge and students passively receiving it, have been the norm for centuries. However, these environments come with their own set of unique challenges that can hinder the learning process for many students.

The One-Size-Fits-All Approach

In a traditional learning environment, it's common for instructors to adopt a uniform teaching approach. This standardization, while helping manage large classrooms, often fails to account for individual learning styles and paces. Consequently, learners who struggle to keep up or those who find the pace too slow might lose interest, leading to disengagement and poor performance.

Limited Interaction and Collaboration

Traditional classrooms often limit student interaction during lessons. The teacher-centric model leaves little room for collaborative learning experiences, which could stifle the development of critical social and communication skills.

Assessment Methods

Traditional education heavily relies on examinations and grades as measures of understanding and success. This approach can lead to a narrow focus on rote-learning and memorization, rather than fostering a deep understanding of the subject matter.

Lack of Real-World Context

In traditional learning environments, there's often a disconnect between what students learn and how these lessons apply to the real world. The focus tends to be on theoretical knowledge, with less emphasis on practical skills and real-world applications.

Strategies to Overcome These Challenges

- **Diversified Teaching Methods:** Incorporating a variety of teaching methods can cater to diverse learning styles. This could include visual aids, hands-on activities, or group discussions.

- **Encourage Interaction:** Promoting active participation in the classroom can foster a more engaging and dynamic learning environment. Interactive activities can stimulate critical thinking and allow students to learn from each other.

- **Holistic Assessments:** Assessments should evaluate more than just recall of information. Including project-based assessments or presentations can provide a more comprehensive understanding of a student's grasp of the topic.

- **Real-World Connections:** Making connections between the curriculum and real-world situations can help students understand the relevance and applicability of their learning.

The Role of Teachers in Addressing These Challenges

Teachers play a critical role in addressing these challenges. By adopting a student-centered approach, teachers can help create a more inclusive, interactive, and effective learning environment. This involves understanding each student's unique needs and strengths, promoting active learning, and providing supportive and constructive feedback.

Advocating for Your Child in School

Navigating the educational system to ensure your child gets the best possible learning experience can be a daunting task. Yet, as parents, it's crucial to be proactive and persistent advocates for your child's academic and social needs. Here's how you can effectively advocate for your child in school.

Understanding Your Child's Needs

Get to know your child's strengths, weaknesses, interests, and challenges. This understanding will guide you in determining what resources and support your child may need in school. Assessments, both academic and behavioral, can provide valuable insights.

Learning About the School System

Educate yourself about your child's school and the broader educational system. Understand the school's policies, procedures, and resources. Familiarize yourself with your rights and responsibilities, and those of your child, under the law.

Building a Positive Relationship with the School

Establish a cooperative relationship with your child's teachers and school administrators. Regular communication and mutual respect can go a long way in resolving issues. Attending parent-teacher meetings and school events can help build these relationships.

Strategies for Effective Advocacy

- **Clear Communication:** Express your concerns clearly and assertively, focusing on your child's needs. Provide specific examples wherever possible.

- **Preparation:** Before meetings, prepare a list of concerns, questions, and potential solutions. This helps to have a focused discussion.

- **Documentation:** Keep records of all communications and meetings. These can be useful for future reference.

- **Collaboration:** Work together with school staff to identify the best strategies and resources for your child.

- **Persistence:** Advocacy is often a long-term effort. Stay committed and persistent, even when faced with setbacks.

When to Seek Outside Help

If your advocacy efforts are not producing the desired results, it might be time to seek outside help. Educational advocates or attorneys can provide guidance and representation, especially when dealing with complex issues like special education services.

While advocating for your child may seem overwhelming at times, remember that you are your child's first and most important advocate. Your active involvement in your child's education can make a significant difference in their academic success and personal growth.

Collaborating with Teachers and School Staff

Building a solid relationship between parents and school staff is an integral part of enhancing a child's educational experience. Collaborating effectively with teachers and school staff not only fosters a supportive learning environment for your child but it also helps you stay informed about your child's progress and challenges.

Understanding the Role of Teachers and School Staff

Teachers are the primary point of contact for your child's academic journey. Other staff members, such as school counselors, administrators, and special education professionals, also play significant roles in shaping your child's school experience. Understanding their roles can provide a framework for effective collaboration.

Building Constructive Relationships

A positive and respectful relationship with your child's teacher is the foundation of successful collaboration. Regularly communicate with them, attend parent-teacher meetings, and participate in school events. Show appreciation for their efforts and maintain an open mind when discussing your child's progress and challenges.

Effective Communication Strategies

- **Be Proactive:** Don't wait for issues to arise before communicating with teachers. Regular check-ins can keep you informed and help prevent minor issues from escalating.

- **Be Clear and Concise:** Clearly articulate your concerns and questions. Provide specific examples to illustrate your points.

- **Listen Actively:** Take time to understand the teacher's perspective. Remember, they interact with your child in a different context and can provide valuable insights.

- **Seek Solutions Together:** Approach conversations with the goal of finding solutions that best support your child's learning.

Collaborating on Special Needs

If your child has special needs, collaboration becomes even more critical. You may need to work closely with special education teachers, school psychologists, and other professionals. Stay involved in the development and implementation of your child's Individualized Education Program (IEP) or 504 plan.

When Disagreements Arise

Disagreements may occur despite your best efforts. If this happens, try to stay calm and focused on the issue at hand. Seek a neutral third party, such as a school counselor or administrator, if you're unable to resolve the disagreement directly.

Collaboration extends beyond addressing issues or challenges. It encompasses working together to enhance your child's overall educational experience. This can include collaborating on enrichment opportunities, discussing your child's social development, and exploring ways to extend learning beyond the classroom.

Individualized Education Plans (IEP) and 504 Plans

Securing supportive academic accommodations is crucial for your son's school success. Two primary tools exist to legally mandate aids and modifications: the 504 Plan and the IEP. As a parent, understanding the difference between these resources is key to accessing the proper help.

What is a 504 Plan?

A 504 Plan refers to Section 504 of the Rehabilitation Act of 1973. It is a document outlining accommodations that a general education student requires to perform on par with peers.

To qualify for a 504 Plan, your child must have a diagnosed disability that impacts major life activities, like:

- Learning

- Concentrating

- Thinking

- Communicating

ADHD would qualify as an eligible condition. The 504 Plan is tailored to the child's needs and is legally binding upon the school to provide.

Common 504 Accommodations

504 Plans grant "reasonable" accommodations so the disability does not limit access to learning. Common accommodations include:

- Extended time on tests and assignments

- Reduced homework or shortened assignments

- Testing in distraction-reduced setting

- Teachers providing class notes or outlines

- Use of a computer for writing tasks

- Seating near the teacher

- Additional time between classes

- Auditory amplification system

- Verbal praise and redirection

The 504 team crafts a personalized plan suited to addressing your son's challenges. Accommodations are adjusted as needs evolve.

The 504 Process

- **Parent referral:** You can request assessment for a 504 Plan at any time. The school must promptly evaluate eligibility.

- **Evaluation:** The school team reviews medical documentation, test scores, teacher observations, and other data to determine impact of the disability on learning.

- **Plan development:** If your child qualifies, a team of teachers, specialists, and yourself develop an appropriate 504 Plan for implementation.

- **Monitoring:** Progress is reviewed periodically. Plans are revised accordingly. 504 Plans are renewed annually.

Unlike an IEP, a 504 Plan does not guarantee particular services, just reasonable accommodations. However, it is useful in providing general education supports.

What is an IEP?

An Individualized Education Plan goes deeper than a 504 Plan in mandating supports. An IEP is for students requiring Special Education services due to a disability affecting learning and academics.

To qualify for an IEP under the Individuals with Disabilities Education Act (IDEA), your child must:

- Have a diagnosed disability like ADHD

- Demonstrate academic skill deficits

- Require Special Education services to access curriculum

The IEP Team

An IEP team consists of:

- The child's parent(s)

- General education teacher

- Special education teacher

- School psychologist

- Administrator

- Specialists like a speech therapist as needed

- The child, when appropriate

This team collaborates to create a legally binding roadmap tailored to the child's needs and goals.

Components of an IEP

An IEP outlines:

- The child's present levels of academic and functional performance

- Annual learning goals

- Special education and related services to be provided

- Percentage of time spent in general vs. special education

- Accommodations and modifications provided in the classroom

- How progress will be tracked and reported

- Transition planning as the child gets older

IEPs are far more comprehensive than 504 Plans in detailing instructional services. They are reviewed and updated annually.

Special Education Services

Special education services are individualized but commonly involve:

- A dedicated special education teacher providing specialized instruction. This may occur one-on-one or in a small group setting.

- Speech therapy, occupational therapy, or other therapies tailored to the child's needs.

- Placement in a special classroom for core subjects like reading or math. Time may be split between special and general education classes.

- Paraprofessional support from an aide providing classroom assistance.

- Transportation services if needed for accessibility.

- Assistive technology like audiobooks, tablets, or memory aids.

The IEP outlines the right amount and types of services to set your child up for academic success.

Getting Started with an IEP

If you believe your son requires Special Education programming:

- Request assessment in writing. The school must promptly determine eligibility and need.

- Provide copies of medical records, past schoolwork, test scores, etc. to establish evidence of his challenges.

- List concerns about your child's academic progress and where he requires extra support.

- Once qualified, provide input collaboratively creating the IEP tailored to his needs.

You are a key member of the IEP team. Do not hesitate to push for services that will support your son's growth. Monitor progress closely and request revisions as needed over time.

Appealing IEP or 504 Decisions

If you disagree with the school's evaluation results or educational plan, you have the right to appeal decisions. Steps include:

- Submitting a written complaint to the school requesting other options.

- Speaking with the school principal if issues are unresolved with the IEP team.

- Requesting mediation between yourself and school representatives.

- Filing for a due process hearing before an impartial officer who will hear both sides and render a legally binding decision.

Hopefully open communication prevents needing formal appeals. But you have recourse to ensure your son receives the programming he requires. Never feel pushed into an IEP or 504 Plan you believe insufficient.

Securing Special Education or 504 Plan services is a pivotal step in managing your son's ADHD at school. These legal mechanisms guarantee aids and programming tailored to his needs. Though navigating the processes takes diligence and persistence, the outcome provides a vital scaffolding for your child's academic journey.

Homework Strategies for Boys with ADHD

Helping a child with Attention Deficit Hyperactivity Disorder (ADHD) can be a challenging task, especially when it comes to homework. The symptoms of ADHD, such as difficulty focusing, forgetfulness, and impulsivity, can make homework time particularly stressful. However, with the right strategies, you can help your child navigate these challenges successfully.

Understanding How ADHD Affects Homework

Children with ADHD often struggle with organization, time management, and concentration - skills that are critical for completing homework. Recognizing how these challenges impact your child's homework process can help you tailor strategies to their specific needs.

Creating a Structured Homework Routine

Routine and structure can provide a sense of security for children with ADHD. Establish a consistent homework schedule, designating a specific start and end time. This provides predictability and helps your child understand what's expected of them.

Setting Up a Conducive Homework Environment

- **Quiet and Distraction-Free:** A quiet, clutter-free area can minimize distractions and help your child focus better.

- **Comfortable and Well-Lit:** Ensure the homework area is comfortable and has adequate lighting.

- **Essential Supplies:** Keep all necessary supplies within reach to prevent your child from having to get up frequently.

Homework Strategies for Boys with ADHD

- **Break Down Tasks:** Large assignments can be overwhelming. Break them down into smaller, manageable tasks.

- **Use Timers:** Timers can help manage attention spans. Encourage your child to work for a set amount of time, then take a short break.

- **Visual Schedules:** Visual aids can be helpful in organizing tasks and keeping track of progress.

- **Positive Reinforcement:** Praise your child's efforts, not just outcomes. Reward progress to motivate your child and boost their self-esteem.

Collaborating with Teachers

Regular communication with your child's teacher can provide valuable insights into your child's academic performance and behavior. Discuss potential accommodations, like extended deadlines or reduced assignments, if necessary.

Seeking Professional Help

If your child continues to struggle with homework despite your best efforts, consider seeking help from a professional. A behavioral therapist or ADHD coach can provide specific strategies and tools tailored to your child's needs.

The Role of Technology in Learning

In the 21st century, technology plays a pivotal role in education. It has transformed the way information is accessed, consumed, and shared, and has opened up a plethora of learning opportunities for students of all ages. However, to harness its full potential, it's essential to understand how technology can best support learning.

Understanding the Relationship Between Technology and Learning

Technology can facilitate personalized and active learning. It provides access to a vast array of resources and enables diverse instructional strategies. However, the key lies in using technology as a tool to enhance learning, not replacing the learning process itself.

Advantages of Technology in Learning

There are several advantages of integrating technology into the learning process:

- **Access to Information:** Technology provides access to a wealth of information and resources, making learning more dynamic and engaging.

- **Personalized Learning:** Learning platforms can adapt to a student's pace and learning style, providing personalized instruction.

- **Collaboration:** Technology facilitates collaboration and communication, allowing students to work together on projects and learn from each other.

- **Skill Development:** The use of technology helps students develop essential skills, such as digital literacy, problem-solving, and critical thinking.

Effective Use of Technology in Learning

While technology offers significant advantages, it's crucial to use it effectively. Here are a few strategies:

- **Integrate Technology Purposefully:** Use technology to enhance learning objectives, not just for the sake of using it.

- **Promote Active Learning:** Encourage students to use technology for research, problem-solving, and creating content.

- **Ensure Digital Literacy:** Teach students how to use technology safely and responsibly.

Challenges and How to Overcome Them

Despite its benefits, the use of technology in learning does pose some challenges:

- **Digital Divide:** Not all students have equal access to technology. Schools and communities should work towards ensuring equitable access to technology and internet services.

- **Screen Time Concerns:** Excessive screen time can have negative health impacts. Balance technology use with offline activities and encourage regular breaks.

- **Online Safety:** Teach students about online safety, privacy, and digital citizenship to guard against potential online risks.

Technology has the power to revolutionize education and create engaging, interactive learning experiences. However, it's essential to remember that technology is just a tool. The effectiveness of its use in learning heavily depends on the strategies employed by educators and the active involvement of students.

Considering Alternative Education Options

When the traditional school system fails to meet a child's needs, exploring alternative options may be the key to academic success. For boys with ADHD who struggle within the constraints of conventional classrooms, a personalized approach can make all the difference. From charter schools to homeschooling and more, consider giving your son an educational environment tailored to how he learns best.

Understanding When to Look Elsewhere

Consider alternative options if your child with ADHD:

- Still performs far below grade level despite accommodations or special education services.

- Suffers severe social difficulties including bullying.

- Experiences extreme anxiety, emotional breakdowns, or refusal to attend school.

- Is facing possible expulsion due to behavioral issues.

- Needs instruction tailored to a particular learning style or interest not offered in traditional schools.

- Has talents better nurtured in a specialized program.

You know your son's needs. If the current system is failing him, trust your instincts and explore choices.

Types of Alternative Education Models

- Charter Schools – Public schools with specialized curriculum, structure, or approaches. Often focused on particular themes like technology, the arts, or project-based learning.

- Private Schools – Offer personalized instruction, very small classes, and highly structured environments catering to children with special needs.

- Online Schools – Use technology to deliver remote instruction virtually. Offer flexible, self-paced options for learning from home.

- Homeschooling – Parents directly provide instruction tailored to the child's needs, schedule, and interests. Allows highly customized education.

- Montessori Schools – Student-directed, hands-on learning environments focused on student interest and developing life skills. Minimal testing and grouping by ability instead of age.

- Special Needs Schools – Specifically serve students with disabilities like ADHD, autism spectrum disorder, dyslexia, etc. with expertise in their needs.

Research options in your area to find the right fit based on your child's needs and learning preferences. Schedule visits to observe firsthand.

Key Features to Look For

Prioritize schools offering:

- Very small class sizes for individualized attention.

- Flexible self-directed learning at their own pace.

- Hands-on, interactive, and movement-based learning activities.

- Arts, music, and creative outlets built into the curriculum.

- Therapies like social skills classes or counseling.

- Sensory spaces for movement breaks.

- Mixed-age classrooms based on ability, not age.

- Outdoor or nature-based learning opportunities.

An alternative program specifically designed for neurodiverse learners like your son with ADHD can make a world of difference.

Questions to Ask When Researching Schools

- How are classes structured on a daily and weekly basis?

- What teaching methods and philosophies are used?

- What training do teachers have for students with special needs?

- What academic and behavioral supports are available?

- What enrichment activities are offered?

- What assistive technology is incorporated?

- How is bullying handled?

- How is student progress tracked and reported?

- How are parents involved in their child's education?

Gathering detailed insights will help determine if the model truly aligns with your son's ideal learning environment.

Pros of Alternative Education

- Individualized instruction focused solely on your child's needs.

- Nurturing, low-stress environments minimizing anxiety.

- Flexible pacing and teaching tailored to their learning style.

- More physical movement and hands-on learning incorporated naturally.

- Opportunity to pursue passions and talents.

- Developing social-emotional skills prioritized alongside academics.

- High teacher-student ratios and specialized support.

The benefits often empower children to excel academically and socially when traditional settings previously failed them.

Potential Cons to Consider

- Possible lack of resources compared to public schools.

- Concerns about limited socialization if classes are very small.

- Potential lack of special education services. Ask about therapies offered.

- No guaranteed continuity year-to-year – programs may change or close unexpectedly.

- Possible gaps in curriculum compared to public schools.

- Potential stigma from others about "different" schooling methods.

Do your due diligence checking credentials,longestablished reputation, and school philosophy when choosing.

Making Alternative Models Work Long-Term

Once enrolled, set your child up for success through:

- Maintaining strong communication with teachers and administrators. Be a partner.

- Providing supplementary learning activities at home to fill any gaps.

- Setting a regular school schedule for consistency even if location changes.

- Having them engage in community or extracurricular activities for social development.

- Working on study and organizational skills not emphasized in alternative programs.

- Being open-minded to tweaking plans over time as needs evolve.

While an alternative program may be a lifeline for your son now, reassess periodically to ensure it continues meeting his needs as he grows. Be willing to switch models if another becomes a better fit.

Overcoming Judgment About Alternative Education

Other parents, teachers, or professionals may pass judgment about "unconventional" schooling. Combat stigma by:

- Advocating confidently for your child's needs. You know him best.

- Explaining how alternative models play to your son's strengths and help him thrive.

- Highlighting academic and social progress made compared to previous school struggles.

- Providing facts on how popular or credible the program is.

- Noting colleges alumni have gone on to attend.

At the end of the day, results and your child's happiness matter far more than other people's opinions. Stay true to what works for your family.

When a child's needs are not being met at their current school, making a change provides hope. Finding an alternative educational approach tailored to your son's learning style and strengths can empower him to success in place of failure. Trust your instincts as his parent to guide him where he will flourish.

CHAPTER 4

DEVELOPING SOCIAL SKILLS AND BUILDING RELATIONSHIPS

Social Challenges for Boys with ADHD

Boys with Attention Deficit Hyperactivity Disorder (ADHD) often face unique social challenges. The symptoms of ADHD, including impulsivity, inattentiveness, and hyperactivity, can make social interactions difficult. Recognizing these challenges and understanding how to address them is crucial for helping boys with ADHD navigate social situations successfully.

Understanding the Social Challenges

Boys with ADHD may struggle with a variety of social issues. These can include difficulty following social norms, reading social cues, or maintaining focus in conversations. They might also act impulsively, leading to behaviors that are seen as disruptive or inappropriate.

Strategies to Help Boys with ADHD Navigate Social Challenges

- **Model Appropriate Social Behavior:** Demonstrating proper social behavior can provide boys with ADHD a clear example to follow.

- **Role-Play Social Situations:** Role-playing can help boys with ADHD practice social interactions in a safe, controlled environment.

- **Teach Emotional Regulation:** Learning to recognize and regulate emotions can be particularly helpful for boys with ADHD, who may struggle with impulsivity.

- **Encourage Participation in Structured Social Activities:** Activities like sports or clubs can provide opportunities for social interaction within a structured environment.

- **Implement Consistent Routines:** Consistency and predictability can help boys with ADHD understand what is expected of them in different social situations.

Collaborating with School and Mental Health Professionals

School can be a challenging environment for boys with ADHD, given the social demands and expectations. Regular communication with teachers and school counselors can help identify potential issues and develop strategies to address them. Additionally, working with mental health professionals, such as psychologists or behavioral therapists, can provide further support.

Fostering Peer Relationships

Helping boys with ADHD build healthy peer relationships can significantly improve their social skills. Encourage playdates, participate in community activities, and provide opportunities for positive social interactions.

Encouraging Healthy Friendships

Meaningful social connections are essential for any child's wellbeing and development. But for boys with ADHD, building and maintaining friendships often proves challenging. Their impulsivity, hyperactivity, and poor emotional control can hinder relating to peers. However, with consistent guidance, you can equip your son with the abilities to nurture rewarding, lasting relationships.

Common Social Struggles for Boys with ADHD

- Impulsiveness causing inappropriate behaviors which alienate peers

- Hyperactivity and noisiness creating social disruption

- Inattention making them seem aloof and uninterested in others

- Difficulty reading social cues, norms, and body language

- Poor concentration impeding following conversations or shared activities

- Low frustration tolerance leading to emotional outbursts

- Fixation on restricted interests not shared by peers

- Aggression or argumentativeness due to poor self-regulation

With support building social competencies, these challenges are surmountable. Arm your son with skills to set him up for connection.

Teaching Friendship Skills through Modeling and Role Play

Explicitly walk through the steps to making and being a good friend:

- How to join group activities and enter conversations politely

- Taking turns talking and avoiding interrupting others

- Asking questions about others' interests to find common ground

- Listening without distraction and making eye contact

- Displaying good sportsmanship during games and competition

- Compromising on activities and handling disappointment maturely

- Expressing empathy for how others feel

- Apologizing after making mistakes or saying hurtful things

Then role play scenarios he may encounter to practice skills. Provide feedback to improve his social toolkit over time.

Practicing Good Conversational Skills

Sustaining dialogues requires concentration boys with ADHD often lack. Have regular back-and-forth chats focusing on:

- Asking questions of the other person

- Limiting rambling on restricted interests

- Maintaining eye contact

- Not interrupting

- Reacting to show interest in what is said

- Sticking to the topic instead of jumping randomly

Praise efforts even if skills are not mastered quickly. With regular rehearsal, conversational abilities will improve.

Finding Common Interests

Shared interests or activities provide social glue. Help your son identify peers who:

- Enjoy similar games, sports, or hobbies

- Appreciate the same funny memes or shows

- Have complementary academic strengths to collaborate

- Attend the same extracurricular activities

Introduce compatible peers through these mutual interests. Having a social anchor will help interactions feel natural rather than forced.

Expanding Friendship Circles

Rather than fixating on one friend, encourage diverse groups through:

- Hosting gatherings with multiple peers to build bonds

- Joining clubs or teams to meet new people

- Practicing entering existing conversations to make connections

- Exchanging contact information to stay in touch

- Nurturing online friendships through gaming or chat groups

Developing an array of friends exposes your son to varied personalities and prevents isolation if one relationship falters.

Handling Teasing and Exclusion

Boys with ADHD are prone to bullying. Help your son counter teasing or exclusion with:

- Appearing confident and unaffected by the taunts

- Using witty humor to deflect the remarks without escalating things

- Saying "No, thank you" firmly and walking away

- Reporting seriously hurtful bullying to trusted adults

Role play comebacks and de-escalation tactics to give him tools for standing up to aggressors while avoiding conflicts spiraling.

Managing Impulsiveness and Hyperactivity

Core ADHD symptoms are friendship repellants if uncontrolled. Set expectations for:

- Not grabbing items impulsively or interrupting constantly

- Remaining seated during conversations instead of jumping around

- Avoiding shouting out random thoughts or comments

- Listening without distraction instead of over-talking

- Speaking at an appropriate volume and distance

Structure activities enabling movement so he can channel hyperactivity constructively while maintaining friendships.

Encouraging Emotional Control

Temper outbursts damage social bonds quickly. Help your son:

- Recognize rising frustration and use calming techniques

- Verbalize anger using "I statements" instead of yelling

- Take a break from friends if upset until composed

- Apologize after calm for hurtful words said in anger

- Explain how ADHD causes emotional reactivity he is working on controlling

Over time, learning to regulate emotions around others will preserve meaningful relationships.

Fostering Reconciliation Skills

Disputes are inevitable. Guide your son through making amends by:

- Taking responsibility for his role without blame

- Sincerely apologizing for actions that hurt or offended

- Listening to the friend's perspective and feelings

- Brainstorming solutions so the issue does not repeat

- Suggesting compensations, like doing nice favors

- Respecting if more time is temporarily needed apart

Developing conflict resolution skills leads to resilient, lasting social bonds.

Helping Make Plans

Impulsiveness causes boys with ADHD to overcommit then forget plans. Provide supports like:

- Recording plans clearly on calendars and setting reminders

- Having him repeat plans back for memory retention

- Confirming commitments the day before get-togethers

- Calling friends when running late or needing to cancel

- Planning hangouts only 1-2 days in advance as capabilities grow

With planning aids in place, he can follow through reliably on peer commitments.

Close friendships boost confidence, provide protective factors against bullying, and build crucial social skills for life. Despite hurdles ADHD may pose, intentionally developing your son's friendship abilities ensures meaningful connections lie ahead.

Building Empathy and Understanding in Your Child

The ability to understand and share others' feelings, known as empathy, is a fundamental human capacity. It fosters positive relationships, promotes social harmony, and drives compassionate action. Cultivating empathy in children from a young age can shape them into caring, understanding individuals and responsible global citizens.

The Importance of Developing Empathy in Children

Empathy enables children to connect with others on a deeper level and appreciate diverse perspectives. It nurtures kindness, reduces bullying, and fosters a sense of inclusion. Additionally, empathetic children are likely to become empathetic adults, contributing to a more compassionate society.

How to Nurture Empathy in Children

Cultivating empathy in children involves deliberate effort and consistent modeling. Here are some strategies:

- **Model Empathetic Behavior:** Children learn by observing their parents. Show empathy to others in your daily interactions.

- **Discuss Emotions:** Regularly talk about feelings and emotions with your child. This can help them better understand their own emotions and those of others.

- **Read Together:** Books can be a fantastic tool for teaching empathy. They allow children to explore different characters' feelings and perspectives.

- **Encourage Perspective-Taking:** Regularly ask your child how they think others might feel in different situations.

- **Promote Kindness and Compassion:** Encourage your child to help others, showing them that their actions can positively impact others.

The Role of Empathy in Conflict Resolution

Empathy can play a vital role in resolving conflicts. By understanding another's perspective, children can address disagreements more effectively and peacefully.

Fostering Empathy in Diverse Social Contexts

Nurturing empathy should extend beyond interpersonal relationships to include diverse social contexts. Encourage your child to consider the experiences of people from different cultures, backgrounds, and abilities.

While fostering empathy is crucial, it's equally important to teach children about boundaries and self-care. They should understand that while being empathetic involves understanding and caring for others' feelings, they should also prioritize their own well-being.

Empathy is not just about understanding others' feelings; it's also about responding with care. It involves taking action to alleviate another person's distress, whether that's through comforting words, a helping hand, or a simple act of kindness. Encourage your child to not only recognize others' emotions but also think about what they can do to help. This active component of empathy, often referred to as "compassionate empathy," can empower your child to make a real difference in their interactions with others.

Navigating Bullying and Peer Pressure

Navigating the complex terrain of social interactions is a crucial part of a child's development. Among these challenges are bullying and peer pressure, both of which can have significant impacts on a child's well-being. Understanding these issues and helping your child to handle them effectively can boost their resilience and self-confidence.

Understanding Bullying and Peer Pressure

Bullying is an aggressive behavior that is intentional and involves an imbalance of power or strength. It can take many forms, such as physical, verbal, relational, or online (cyberbullying). Peer pressure, on the other hand, is the influence that a peer group, observers or individual exerts, causing others to change their attitudes, values, or behaviors to conform to group norms.

Strategies to Handle Bullying

- **Open Communication:** Encourage your child to talk about their school life and friendships. Be a good listener and provide a safe, non-judgmental space for them.

- **Recognize the Signs:** Changes in mood, behavior, or physical appearance can be signs of bullying. Keep an eye out for any sudden changes.

- **Teach Assertiveness:** Empower your child to stand up for themselves. Teach them to voice their feelings without resorting to aggression.

- **Involve School Authorities:** If your child is being bullied at school, involve teachers and school administrators. They can help enforce anti-bullying policies and ensure your child's safety.

Strategies to Handle Peer Pressure

- **Build Self-Esteem:** A strong sense of self can help your child resist negative peer pressure. Reinforce their strengths and unique qualities.

- **Teach Decision-Making Skills:** Help your child learn to make informed decisions based on their values, not on what others are doing.

- **Discuss Scenarios:** Talk about different peer pressure scenarios and brainstorm appropriate responses.

- **Choose Friends Wisely:** Encourage your child to choose friends who respect their choices and do not exert negative influence.

Cultivating a Supportive Environment

Establishing a supportive home environment is crucial. Your child should feel comfortable discussing their concerns and know that they can rely on your support.

Bullying and peer pressure can be daunting, but they can also serve as opportunities to build resilience and assertiveness. Ensure your child understands that it's okay to seek help and that they don't have to deal with these challenges alone.

Coaching Your Child for Social Success

Navigating social situations can feel like an obstacle course for children with ADHD. Impulsivity, emotional dysregulation, and difficulty reading social cues put them at a disadvantage among peers. However, with consistent coaching from you, your son can gain the skills needed to socially thrive. Think of yourself as a sports coach, providing ongoing training, support, and cheerleading on the sidelines.

Lay the Foundation with Social Stories

Use illustrations and short narratives to teach expected behaviors for various social scenarios like:

- How to have a back-and-forth conversation

- Keeping hands to self when excited

- Waiting turns patiently when playing games

- Saying please and thank you

- Following the rules of a group activity

Read stories together frequently and have your child recount key lessons. The more exposure through repetition, the better their comprehension.

Run Through Play "Drills"

Set up role play scenarios to rehearse target skills:

- Taking turns sharing toys or talking

- Losing a game gracefully without outbursts

- Responding politely when someone makes a mistake

- Introducing themselves confidently to new people

- Apologizing for bumping into someone accidentally

Model expected behaviors first. Then observe your child practicing and provide warm, corrective feedback to refine their technique.

Schedule Regular Skill "Scrimmages"

Have your child interact in controlled social situations to flex their developing abilities.

- Invite a patient friend over for a playdate.

- Enroll in a group lesson for an activity he enjoys.

- Gather two families at a park and let kids play while you supervise.

The more "scrimmage" reps your child gets, the more instinctive applying skills becomes when performance counts.

Help Them Suit Up with Coping Strategies

Equip your player for moments of difficulty with handy coping methods:

- Taking deep breaths when frustrated

- Counting to 10 silently before reacting

- Going to a quiet space when overwhelmed

- Squeezing a stress ball in their pocket

- Looking to you for an encouraging nod

Just like star athletes rely on sports psychologists, children with ADHD need tools to center themselves when challenges arise.

Review the Playbook Regularly

Keep key lessons front and center by:

- Rereading favorite social stories often

- Posting visual behavior reminders around the house

- Role playing especially difficult situations

- Practicing coping methods before events

Frequent review strengthens their comprehension and recall when applied in real time.

Help Expand Their Team

Guide your child in making new supportive friendships:

- Pair them with a buddy for group activities

- Facilitate playdates with patient peers

- Encourage joining clubs or teams around shared interests

Surrounding your player with a solid team boosts confidence during the game.

Provide a Halftime Pep Talk When Needed

If your child gets overwhelmed or acts out during a social activity, step aside for a quick regroup:

- Offer empathy while reviewing what went wrong

- Brainstorm a plan to improve behavior moving forward

- Provide an encouraging pep talk emphasizing their capabilities

- Remind them of helpful coping methods

- Highlight past successes as proof they can handle this

This motivational timeout helps them take a deep breath and get back in the game.

Model Good Sportsmanship

Children imitate the behaviors they see from coaches. Be mindful to:

- Stay calm and polite even when frustrated

- Offer praise far more than criticism

- Admit mistakes and apologize for overreactions

- Use "I statements" when addressing problems

- Remain patient but firm in upholding rules

Your example is their most powerful training guide.

Help Them Bounce Back from Losses

Don't reprimand losing their cool; emotions are part of the sport. Instead:

- Acknowledge feelings are normal when things go wrong

- Discuss what triggered the reaction and better choices next time

- Note skills they applied well despite the setback

- Remind them all players lose sometimes – it's part of learning

With your empathetic support, they will grow more resilient.

Celebrate Wins, However Small

Highlight every forward stride!

- Cheer reaching short-term goals

- Post trophies (certificates) displaying progress

- Share successes proudly with other caring adults

Recognizing advancement motivates athletes to keep training and building skill sets.

Coaching your child towards social success requires dedication, positivity, and teamwork. With active preparation and practice, they can gain the confidence and abilities to thrive on the playing field. Expect setbacks but focus on instilling a love of the growth process. Your unwavering support as their biggest fan will give them strength to shine.

ADHD and the Family Dynamic

The diagnosis of Attention Deficit Hyperactivity Disorder (ADHD) in a child can significantly influence the family dynamic. It introduces unique challenges that can impact relationships, routines, and overall family functioning. However, with understanding, patience, and strategic approaches, families can navigate these challenges and create a supportive environment that fosters the child's growth and development.

Understanding ADHD

ADHD is a neurodevelopmental disorder characterized by inattention, impulsivity, and hyperactivity. It affects a child's ability to focus, follow instructions, and control impulses. Understanding these characteristics is the first step in adapting the family dynamic.

Influences on the Family Dynamic

ADHD can impact the family dynamic in various ways. Parents might feel stressed or overwhelmed by their child's behaviors, siblings might feel neglected, and the child with ADHD might feel misunderstood. Recognizing these impacts is crucial for addressing them effectively.

Strategies for Managing the Family Dynamic

Several strategies can help manage the family dynamic when a child has ADHD:

- **Education and Understanding:** Ensure all family members understand ADHD. This fosters empathy and reduces misconceptions.

- **Establish Routines:** Consistent routines can help a child with ADHD understand expectations and promote a sense of security.

- **Positive Reinforcement:** Recognize and reward positive behaviors. This encourages your child to repeat them.

- **Clear Communication:** Use simple, clear instructions when communicating with your child.

- **Professional Support:** Don't hesitate to seek support from psychologists, educators, and support groups.

The Role of Parents

Parents play a critical role in managing the family dynamic. It's essential to stay patient, maintain a positive outlook, and model appropriate behaviors.

The Role of Siblings

Siblings can provide support, but they may also need support themselves. Ensure they feel heard and valued, and encourage positive interactions between siblings.

While it's essential to address the unique challenges associated with ADHD, it's equally important to celebrate the strengths it can bring. Children with ADHD often exhibit creativity, enthusiasm, and a unique perspective on the world. Harnessing these strengths can bring a positive dynamic to the family.

CHAPTER 5

ADHD TREATMENT OPTIONS

Behavioral Therapy: Techniques and Benefits

Behavioral therapy represents a broad category of therapeutic interventions designed to change maladaptive or unhealthy behaviors. Rooted in the principles of learning theory, these techniques have profound implications in helping individuals overcome a variety of psychological disorders, such as anxiety, depression, ADHD, and more.

Understanding Behavioral Therapy

Behavioral Therapy is based on the premise that behaviors are learned and can therefore be unlearned or reformed. It focuses less on the underlying root causes of behaviors and more on changing the behaviors themselves.

Core Techniques of Behavioral Therapy

There are several techniques used in behavioral therapy, each tailored to address specific types of behavioral challenges:

- **Cognitive Behavioral Therapy (CBT):** This form of therapy combines behavioral therapy with cognitive therapy. It is focused on changing thought patterns that lead to maladaptive behaviors.

- **Dialectical Behavior Therapy (DBT):** A type of CBT, DBT is often used for individuals with severe personality disorders. It focuses on accepting uncomfortable thoughts, feelings, or behaviors instead of struggling with them.

- **Exposure Therapy:** This technique is often used to treat phobias and anxiety disorders. It involves exposing individuals to the source of their fear or anxiety in a controlled, safe environment.

- **Systematic Desensitization:** This method involves gradually exposing individuals to a feared situation or object, starting with the least fearful and progressing to the most fearful.

Benefits of Behavioral Therapy

Behavioral therapy offers numerous benefits:

- **Effectiveness:** Numerous studies have shown the effectiveness of behavioral therapy in treating a variety of psychological disorders.

- **Versatility:** The techniques can be adapted for individuals of all ages and for various disorders.

- **Skill Development:** Behavioral therapy provides individuals with practical strategies and skills to manage their behaviors.

- **Improved Quality of Life:** By addressing and changing maladaptive behaviors, individuals can improve their overall quality of life.

The Role of the Therapist in Behavioral Therapy

The therapist's role in behavioral therapy is to guide the individual through the process of behavior change. They provide a safe space for individuals to explore their behaviors, challenge their thoughts, and learn new strategies.

The Role of the Individual in Behavioral Therapy

The individual plays an active role in behavioral therapy. They are encouraged to explore their behaviors, challenge their thought patterns, and apply new strategies in their daily lives.

Understanding Medication Options

Medication is commonly used alongside behavioral interventions as part of a comprehensive treatment plan for ADHD. For many boys, medication can be life-changing in curbing hyperactive and impulsive symptoms while improving focus. As a parent, arming yourself with knowledge about available pharmaceutical options helps ensure an informed decision about what is best for your individual child.

How ADHD Medications Work

ADHD medications alter brain chemical messengers (neurotransmitters) to:

- Increase ability to focus and reduce distractibility

- Improve organization and motivation

- Decrease excessive movement and fidgeting

- Enable greater emotional regulation and impulse control

This allows boys to pursue tasks with sustained attention and reduced behavioral issues.

Common Types of ADHD Medications

- **Stimulants:** First-line medications that increase dopamine signals in the brain. Allow improved concentration and reduced hyperactivity. Examples include methylphenidate (Ritalin) and amphetamine/dextroamphetamine (Adderall).

- **Non-Stimulants:** Treat ADHD by different mechanisms without stimulation. Used if stimulants cause side effects or are ineffective. Examples are atomoxetine (Strattera), clonidine (Kapvay), and guanfacine (Intuniv).

- **Antidepressants:** Sometimes prescribed alongside stimulants to target both ADHD and co-occurring anxiety or depression. Examples are fluoxetine (Prozac) and sertraline (Zoloft).

Medication Options by Release Method

Stimulant and non-stimulant medications come in different forms that impact duration:

- **Short-Acting:** Effects last about 4 hours. Taken 2-3 times per day.

- **Intermediate-Acting:** Effects last 8-10 hours so taken twice daily.

- **Long-Acting/Extended Release:** Effects last 10-12+ hours so taken once each morning.

- **Liquid Solutions:** Absorbed quickly into the bloodstream.

- **Skin Patches:** Applied once daily releasing medication transdermally.

- **Capsule Form:** Varying release times depending on capsule composition.

Discuss options with your doctor to determine which release method best fits your child's daily schedule and needs.

Key Medication Considerations

- Effectiveness - Does it sufficiently improve target ADHD symptoms?

- Duration - How long do effects last? Will multiple daily doses be needed?

- Side Effects - What potential adverse effects should be monitored?

- Interactions - Does it interact with any other medications or supplements?

- Cost - How expensive is the medication? Is insurance coverage or financial assistance available?

- Administration - Can your child easily swallow pills or prefer a liquid, patch, or capsule?

- Preference - Does your child have concerns or preferences about medication type or method?

Weigh priorities like efficacy, convenience, and affordability when making decisions.

Optimizing Medication Results

Follow these best practices:

- Take medication consistently - Avoid forgotten or skipped doses.

- Track symptoms/side effects - Note effectiveness over time at follow-up appointments.

- Communicate openly - Share concerns and updates with your doctor.

- Use reminders - Set phone alarms for doses.

- Eliminate vitamin C before doses - It reduces absorption.

- Give at the same times daily - Routinize for consistency.

- Store properly - Avoid heat, humidity, or dampness.

Adhering to the treatment regimen helps maximize benefit.

Monitoring Side Effects

Common potential side effects to watch for include:

- Decreased appetite - Your child may not feel hungry, especially at first. Monitor nutrition.

- Trouble sleeping - Adjust timing so medication wears off sufficiently before bedtime.

- Headaches, stomachaches - Generally dissipate within a few weeks once the body adjusts.

- Mood changes - Irritability or emotional reactivity could increase initially.

- Tics - Monitor for any unusual repetitive movements or vocal sounds.

Notify your doctor immediately if any serious or prolonged side effects emerge. Tweaking timing or dosage often helps.

Weighing Medication Holidays

Long-term "medication holidays" are usually not recommended. However, some families opt to take short breaks during low-demand times like summer or holidays. Potential pros include:

- Assessing how their ADHD symptoms function without medication

- Observing side effects like poor appetite or sleep issues

- Allowing the body to "reset" and avoid building tolerance

- Making medication feel less permanent or stigmatized

If you choose to pursue medication holidays, collaborate closely with your child's doctor on timing and return plans. Consistency is key for most kids.

Transitioning Off Medication

For some children, ADHD medication is needed long-term into adulthood. For others, doctors recommend transitioning off during adolescence once behavior regulation improves.

Signs a child may be ready for a trial without medication include:

- Minimal ADHD symptoms present for an extended time

- Utilizing behavioral strategies successfully unprompted

- Displaying emotional maturity and impulse control

- Achieving stable academic performance

- Experiencing major side effects negatively impacting health

Work closely with your doctor and let teachers know if you conduct a trial period without medication. Restarting is always an option if challenges return.

In summary, weigh medication options thoughtfully as part of your son's overall ADHD management. While not right for all children, for many the benefits significantly outweigh the risks when mindfully monitored. Partner closely with your son's pediatrician to make the most informed choice about whether medication is appropriate.

The Role of Diet and Exercise

Fostering a healthy lifestyle involves a holistic approach that encompasses both diet and exercise. These two elements form a symbiotic relationship, each reinforcing and amplifying the effects of the other. Together, they can significantly influence health outcomes, enhancing physical well-being, mental health, and overall quality of life.

Understanding the Importance of Diet

The food we consume plays a crucial role in how we feel, how effectively our body functions, and our susceptibility to certain health conditions. A balanced diet, rich in essential nutrients, fuels our body, supports our immune system, and promotes overall health.

1. **Energy Provision:** Food provides the energy required for bodily functions and physical activities.

2. **Nutrient Supply:** A balanced diet ensures an adequate supply of essential nutrients like vitamins, minerals, proteins, healthy fats, and carbohydrates.

3. **Disease Prevention:** A nutrient-rich diet can help prevent various health conditions, including heart disease, diabetes, obesity, and certain types of cancer.

Understanding the Importance of Exercise

Regular exercise is another cornerstone of a healthy lifestyle. It strengthens the body, improves mood, boosts energy levels, and can ward off a host of health problems.

- **Physical Health:** Exercise enhances cardiovascular health, strengthens muscles, improves flexibility, and boosts metabolism.

- **Mental Health:** Regular physical activity can alleviate symptoms of depression and anxiety, enhance mood, improve sleep, and boost self-esteem.

- **Disease Prevention:** Exercise can help prevent and manage a range of health problems, including heart disease, high blood pressure, and type 2 diabetes.

Integrating Diet and Exercise

Diet and exercise are most effective when integrated. A well-balanced diet supports physical activity by providing the necessary energy and nutrients, while regular exercise can help manage weight and maintain a healthy appetite.

- **Plan Balanced Meals:** Incorporate a variety of nutrient-rich foods into your meals, including fruits, vegetables, lean proteins, whole grains, and healthy fats.

- **Stay Hydrated:** Water plays a key role in nutrient transportation and body temperature regulation, especially during exercise.

- **Regular and Consistent Exercise:** Aim for at least 150 minutes of moderate-intensity or 75 minutes of high-intensity exercise per week.

- **Listen to Your Body:** Pay attention to your body's signals. Rest when you need to and adjust your diet and exercise routine as needed.

Embarking on a journey towards a healthier lifestyle involves making conscious decisions about what you eat and how you move. Remember, the aim is not perfection, but consistency. Gradual, sustainable changes are more effective and long-lasting than drastic, short-term measures.

Alternative Therapies: Neurofeedback, Mindfulness, and More

Navigating the maze of health and wellness can be challenging. Conventional approaches, while effective, may not always offer complete solutions. This is where alternative therapies like neurofeedback, mindfulness, and others step in, complementing traditional methods and offering holistic ways to enhance well-being.

Demystifying Neurofeedback

Neurofeedback is a non-invasive form of therapy that involves training the brain to function more efficiently. It uses real-time displays of brain activity to teach self-regulation of brain function.

- **What is Neurofeedback?** Neurofeedback, or EEG biofeedback, uses electroencephalography (EEG) to monitor brain wave patterns and provide feedback. This feedback helps individuals learn to regulate their own brain waves, leading to improved mental performance and well-being.

- **Benefits of Neurofeedback:** Neurofeedback can aid in managing a variety of conditions, including ADHD, anxiety, depression, sleep disorders, and migraines. It's also used to improve cognitive performance and stress management.

- **Getting Started with Neurofeedback:** Neurofeedback should be performed under the guidance of a trained professional. During sessions, sensors are placed on the scalp to measure brainwave activity. The feedback from these measurements is displayed on a screen, which the individual uses to learn how to control their brainwaves.

Exploring Mindfulness

Mindfulness is a psychological process that involves bringing one's attention to experiences occurring in the present moment. It encourages you to slow down, be aware of your surroundings and your feelings, and accept them without judgment.

- **Understanding Mindfulness:** Mindfulness is about being fully engaged in the here and now. It involves focusing on your senses and observing without judgment.

- **Benefits of Mindfulness:** Regular practice of mindfulness can reduce stress, improve emotional regulation, increase self-awareness, and enhance life satisfaction. It has also been shown to have positive effects on physical health, including improved immune function and lower blood pressure.

- **Practicing Mindfulness:** Mindfulness can be practiced in many ways. It can involve formal practices like meditation and yoga, or informal practices like mindful eating or walking. The key is to find a practice that suits your lifestyle and preferences.

Discovering Other Alternative Therapies

Apart from neurofeedback and mindfulness, there are several other alternative therapies that can contribute to overall well-being.

- **Yoga:** A mind-body practice that combines physical postures, breathing exercises, meditation, and ethical principles.

- **Acupuncture:** An ancient form of Chinese medicine that involves inserting thin needles into specific points on the body.

- **Aromatherapy:** The use of aromatic essential oils to improve physical and emotional well-being.

Always remember to seek professional guidance before embarking on any new therapy. What works for one person may not work for another, so it's essential to find the right approach that suits your individual needs and preferences.

While alternative therapies offer a myriad of benefits, it's important not to view them as a replacement for traditional healthcare. Instead, think of them as tools that can complement and enhance your overall treatment plan. It's about creating a bespoke approach to health and wellness that encompasses all aspects of your life.

Making the Best Treatment Choice for Your Child

With a range of behavioral, educational, and medical interventions available, choosing the right ADHD treatment plan can feel overwhelming as a parent. However, by thoroughly understanding your child's unique symptom presentation, weighing pros and cons of options, and collaborating with a multidisciplinary team, you can craft an individualized management strategy. Factors like age, symptom severity, side effects, and family circumstances all play a role in determining the ideal mix of therapies.

Assembling Your Child's ADHD Support Team

First, build a knowledgeable care team including:

- Your child's primary pediatrician to diagnose ADHD and prescribe medication if desired. Oversee treatment plan.

- A psychologist for behavioral assessments and therapy.

- Teachers providing academic support and classroom accommodations.

- Other school specialists like counselors, occupational therapists, or speech therapists as needed.

- Family members willing to help implement strategies at home.

This combination of medical, psychological, educational, and familial support provides comprehensive insight into your child's needs.

Understanding the Full Picture

To make informed treatment decisions, identify:

- Primary ADHD symptoms impacting functioning

- ADHD presentation - inattentive, hyperactive, or combined type

- Co-occurring conditions like anxiety, learning disabilities etc.

- Severity level - mild, moderate or severe

- Current lifestyle factors, stressors, and family dynamic

- Your child's preferences and concerns about treatment

The full context shapes what combination and intensity of interventions is required. There is no universal plan.

Common ADHD Management Components

- Behavior Modification Therapy - Structure, routines, reward systems

- Classroom Accommodations - IEP or 504 plan services

- Parenting Strategies - Clear communication, emotional support

- Social Skills Training - For improved peer interactions

- Psychotherapy - Targeting emotional regulation or self-esteem

- Organization and Study Skills - To strengthen executive functioning

- ADHD Medication - Stimulant or non-stimulant prescription

- Alternative Therapies - Diet changes, supplements, biofeedback

Evaluate components most critical for your child's needs and development phase. Multimodal care is ideal.

Setting Treatment Goals

Define target outcomes like:

- Improving concentration and on-task behavior

- Reducing impulsiveness and hyperactivity

- Strengthening emotional regulation

- Building positive social skills and friendships

- Boosting academic achievement and learning skills

- Improving home structure, routines and relationships

Well-defined goals allow measuring progress and effectiveness in both the short and long-term. Revisit them at regular intervals.

Assessing Benefits and Side Effects

Carefully monitor each component's efficacy and any side effects:

- Note symptom improvements targeting goals.

- Record side effects like insomnia, appetite changes, mood changes, headaches etc.

- Measure academic and/or social functioning improvements.

- Ask your child's perspective on progress and comfort with treatments.

Frequently sharing observations with your support team allows optimizing the plan.

Adjusting the Treatment Plan

Be prepared to fine-tune approaches over time as:

- Your child's ADHD symptoms evolve with age and development

- Certain interventions prove more or less helpful

- Side effects emerge requiring change

- Family schedule or ability to adhere to plan shifts

- Other parental concerns or priorities arise

Remain flexible. Make changes to keep treatments aligned with your child's needs.

Finding the Right Medication if Desired

If choosing medication:

- Start with stimulant class for optimal ADHD relief.

- Note effects on focus, hyperactivity, emotions, appetite, sleep.

- Adjust dose amount slowly as needed.

- Change to non-stimulant class if side effects are prohibitive.

- Utilize different delivery methods - extended release or patches.

Finding the most effective ADHD medication with minimal side effects often requires persistence and trial-and-error.

Supplementing at Home

Support therapies through:

- Maintaining structure/routines. Use visual schedules.

- Providing movement and sensory breaks.

- Teaching organizational/planning skills. Use checklists and reminders.

- Encouraging healthy habits - nutrition, exercise, sleep.

- Fostering social connections through playdates or clubs.

Consistency across school and home boosts skill development.

Incorporating Your Child's Voice

Empower your child by:

- Explaining treatment choices using age-appropriate language

- Addressing their concerns and preferences

- Eliciting input on goals and progress

- Respecting hesitations or discomfort

- Giving options for involvement where possible

Your partnership increases motivation and success.

Crafting an optimal ADHD management plan is an ongoing collaboration between you, your child, and your support team. With careful observation, flexibility, patience, and tweaking, you will dial in targeted strategies for thriving at home, school, and socially. Stay hopeful - with the right mix of care, an ADHD diagnosis does not limit your child's potential.

CHAPTER 6

EMPOWERING YOUR CHILD: BUILDING INDEPENDENCE AND RESILIENCE

Teaching Your Child Self-Advocacy

In the journey of life, few skills are as vital as self-advocacy. It's the ability to assert oneself, to express one's needs and rights effectively, and to make informed decisions. For children, developing this skill is crucial as it enables them to navigate the world with confidence, resilience, and independence.

Understanding Self-Advocacy in Children

Self-advocacy involves understanding one's rights and interests, communicating them effectively, and making decisions to promote one's well-being. For children, it's about learning to speak up for themselves, ask for what they need, and make choices that align with their values and goals.

- **What is Self-Advocacy?** At its core, self-advocacy is about taking charge of one's life. It involves standing up for oneself, taking responsibility, and being proactive.

- **Why is Self-Advocacy Important?** Developing self-advocacy skills can empower children to navigate social, academic, and professional environments more effectively. It fosters independence, builds confidence, and encourages problem-solving.

Cultivating Self-Advocacy Skills in Your Child

Teaching self-advocacy is not a one-time event, but a gradual, ongoing process. It involves fostering a supportive environment, providing opportunities for practice, and modeling effective self-advocacy.

- **Encourage Open Communication:** Cultivate an atmosphere where your child feels safe expressing their thoughts, feelings, and needs. Regularly engage in open-ended conversations that encourage your child to share.

- **Model Self-Advocacy:** Show your child what it looks like to stand up for oneself. Share instances where you've had to advocate for yourself and explain how you navigated the situation.

- **Teach Them Their Rights:** Educate your child about their rights and responsibilities. This can empower them to make informed decisions and stand up for themselves when necessary.

- **Foster Problem-Solving Skills:** Encourage your child to identify problems, think of possible solutions, and make decisions. This can help them become more proactive and resourceful.

Guiding Your Child in Real-Life Situations

When it comes to teaching self-advocacy, real-life scenarios serve as excellent learning opportunities. These instances can help your child apply the skills they've learned in a practical context.

- **School Situations:** Encourage your child to communicate with teachers about their learning needs. They could ask for clarification on assignments, request extra help, or express concerns about classroom dynamics.

- **Social Interactions:** Guide your child in asserting themselves in social situations. They could express their feelings when a friend upsets them, or ask for a turn during a game.

- **Medical Appointments:** Allow your child to speak for themselves during medical appointments. They could explain their symptoms to the doctor, ask questions about their treatment, or express any fears or concerns they may have.

As parents, it can be challenging to step back and let our children advocate for themselves. It's natural to want to step in and solve problems for them. However, by doing so, we may inadvertently inhibit the development of their self-advocacy skills. It's essential to provide guidance and support while still allowing them to take the lead.

No two children are alike, and neither are their paths to self-advocacy. Some children may naturally be more assertive, while others may need more encouragement and practice. It's vital to be patient, provide positive reinforcement, and celebrate your child's victories, no matter how small.

Developing Problem-Solving Skills

When met with a roadblock, some people freeze, some retreat, and some navigate around it. Those who choose the latter have mastered an invaluable skill: problem-solving. The ability to face challenges head-on, analyze them, and take effective action is not just beneficial—it's essential. It enables us to deal with complexities in all areas of life, from personal to professional.

Understanding Problem-Solving

Problem-solving is a structured approach to addressing an issue or challenge. It involves identifying the problem, analyzing potential solutions, making a decision, and evaluating the outcome.

- **What is Problem-Solving?** Problem-solving is a mental process that involves discovering, analyzing, and solving problems. The ultimate goal of problem-solving is to overcome obstacles and find a solution that resolves the issue.

- **Why is Problem-Solving Essential?** The ability to solve problems is a vital skill in daily life, education, and employment. It fosters resilience, creativity, and critical thinking. It also promotes adaptability, an essential trait in our ever-changing world.

Developing Problem-Solving Skills

Cultivating problem-solving skills is a layered process. It involves practicing critical thinking, nurturing creativity, and learning from experience.

- **Foster Critical Thinking:** Critical thinking involves analyzing information objectively and making a reasoned judgment. Encourage reflective thinking, questioning assumptions, and considering multiple perspectives.

- **Encourage Creativity:** Creative thinking can lead to innovative solutions. Promote activities that stimulate creativity, such as brainstorming, mind mapping, or free writing.

- **Value Mistakes as Learning Opportunities:** Mistakes are often seen as failures, but they are valuable for learning. When a solution doesn't work out, use it as an opportunity to analyze what went wrong and how it can be improved.

Practicing Problem-Solving Techniques

There are numerous strategies for problem-solving. Here are a few classic methods:

- **Brainstorming:** This technique involves generating a list of ideas without judgment or analysis. It encourages creative thinking and can often lead to innovative solutions.

- **The Five Whys:** This technique involves asking "Why?" five times to get to the root cause of a problem. It's a simple but powerful tool for uncovering the underlying issues.

- **SWOT Analysis:** This method involves examining the Strengths, Weaknesses, Opportunities, and Threats related to a problem or decision. It provides a comprehensive view of the situation and can guide the choice of solution.

- **Decision Matrix:** This tool involves listing all possible solutions and their associated factors, then scoring each one to determine the best option. It helps to make decisions based on a systematic analysis of all possibilities.

Real-world application of these techniques and the experience gained from their usage will gradually build your problem-solving acumen. Remember, problem-solving is like a muscle—the more you use it, the stronger it gets.

While developing problem-solving skills, it's crucial to maintain a positive, solution-focused mindset. Challenges are a part of life, and viewing them as opportunities for growth rather than insurmountable obstacles can make a significant difference. This approach, known as a growth mindset, can enhance problem-solving abilities and lead to better outcomes.

Encouraging Responsibility and Accountability

Taking responsibility for their actions and being held accountable for meeting expectations are skills that don't come naturally to boys with ADHD. Their executive functioning challenges make it difficult to connect choices with consequences. However, teaching personal accountability in an empathetic, constructive way helps boys learn to self-manage their behaviors and contributions.

Why Responsibility is Difficult

Boys with ADHD struggle with responsibility because:

- Impulsivity causes acting without thinking.

- Distractibility leads to forgetting tasks or instructions.

- Disorganization hampers tracking assignments.

- Hyperfocus derails preparing for upcoming obligations.

- Difficulty estimating time results in lateness or missed deadlines.

- Lower frustration tolerance leads to giving up easily.

Adjust expectations while scaffolding skills development. Accountability comes gradually.

Ways to Encourage Personal Responsibility

- Frame it positively - take pride in being reliable.

- Use checklists and reminders to support follow-through.

- Have them repeat instructions back when assigning a task.

- Celebrate effort toward responsibility, even if imperfect.

- Share examples of how responsibility helps gain others' trust.

- Involve them in solving lapses - "What could you do differently next time?"

- Balance freedom with accountability as skills improve.

Emphasize capability over perfection. Self-regulation takes practice.

Using Accountability Systems

External motivators like rewards or consequences can teach accountability. Possible systems include:

- Homework or chore charts with stickers for completion

- Point/token systems redeemable for prizes

- Logical consequences related to the task (e.g. incomplete homework means no playtime)

- Clear warnings if expectations are not met before enforcing consequences

- Removal of privileges temporarily if warranted

- Verbal praise and recognition for progress made

Be consistent applying agreed-upon systems. Evolve approaches as needed based on your child's development.

Assigning Age-Appropriate Responsibilities

Match assigned duties to your son's abilities:

- **Toddlers:** Simple self-care tasks like dressing themselves or toy clean up. Use visual aids.

- **Preschoolers:** Daily routines like feeding a pet, putting away their laundry, or watering plants. Use checklists.

- **Elementary:** Focus on schoolwork and household chores like taking out trash or doing dishes. Provide reminders.

- **Tweens:** Ensuring homework is completed independently and maintaining their living space. Track with apps if helpful.

- **Teens:** Part-time jobs, managing schedules, driving responsibly, planning for the future. Provide coaching as needed.

Checklists, alarms, and supervision help instill habits over time.

Teaching Task Planning Skills

Breaking down tasks improves organization and follow-through. Model steps like:

- Clarifying instructions and writing them down

- Identifying materials needed

- Estimating time required

- Scheduling task completion among other commitments

- Setting a timer or alarm for a reminder

- Checking work afterward for errors

- Communicating completion

Task analysis strengthens executive functioning over time.

Encouraging Responsibility with Money

Managing allowances and finances builds accountability. Consider:

- Giving small commission for completed chores.

- Requiring saving a portion of gift money received.

- Providing an allowance to budget for wants.

- Having them track expenditures and balance savings.

- Helping them open a bank account to monitor balances.

- Explaining responsible spending and saving habits.

- Only purchasing wants if they contribute their own money.

- Loaning larger purchases they repay from allowance over time.

Financial responsibility skills prepare them for increasing independence.

Accepting Consequences of Irresponsibility

When lapses occur, avoid anger. Calmly review how the mistake resulted from action (or inaction) and now requires accountability. Example: "You did not finish your homework because you chose to play video games instead. That means you will get a zero for the assignment." Allow natural outcomes to reinforce personal responsibility.

Empowering Responsible Decision-Making

- Frame choices as "if-then" scenarios - "If you finish your homework first, then you can play."

- Discuss how decisions affect themselves and others.

- Guide resolving poor choices independently before intervening.

- Praise thoughtful decision-making, not just outcomes.

- Let small choices build empowerment over time.

Boys gain confidence handling responsibility when given space to self-correct with support.

Owning and Managing ADHD Challenges

Your son should take an active role managing ADHD by:

- Voicing symptoms honestly with doctors so treatment is effective.

- Using medications and therapies responsibly if prescribed.

- Monitoring effectiveness and side effects of treatments.

- Researching ADHD to better self-advocate and educate others.

- Identifying when support is needed and seeking it proactively.

- Tracking assignments and schedules independently.

- Building skills to compensate for difficulties.

Intentionally developing accountability and maturity around ADHD cultivates resilience.

Responsibility requires ongoing coaching for boys with ADHD but pays lifelong dividends in self-confidence, resilience, and independence. Maintain compassion about struggles while fostering accountability. With scaffolding, your son will gain the skills to take the reins.

Celebrating Wins and Coping with Setbacks

Raising a child with ADHD is filled with peaks and valleys. Their neurodiversity leads to illogical emotional swings, scattered focus, forgetfulness, and impulse-control challenges. However, as a parent you play a vital role in shaping how your son perceives these setbacks and accomplishments along the way. Maintaining unwavering positivity and support through ups and downs teaches resilience and emotional maturity.

The Power of Praise

Sincere, specific praise is invaluable for boys who may hear far more correction than encouragement in their day-to-day life due to ADHD-related behaviors. Catch your son doing good and let him know it!

- Celebrate effort and persistence towards goals, not just end results. The path to achievement matters.

- Recognize small wins, like getting ready for school without a battle. Progress can be incremental.

- Cheer competencies and strengths he demonstrates in academics, sports, music or social interactions.

- Use descriptive language like "I am so proud of how focused you were solving that math problem!" to reinforce behaviors.

Heighten awareness of the link between his efforts and accomplishments to motivate positive change.

Throwing Confetti for Milestones

Major developmental milestones or special achievements deserve a big celebration.

- Make a custom certificate he can hang up highlighting the skill or success.

- Have a special family dinner or dessert in his honor.

- Call special relatives to share the proud news.

- Give sincere accolades in a written letter.

- Commemorate with photos.

- Plan a fun experience like a trip to celebrate.

- Display mementos like ribbons or trophies prominently.

Commemorating significant milestones helps cement self-confidence.

Reframing Setbacks as Opportunities

The impulsivity and distractibility accompanying ADHD means setbacks will happen frequently. When missteps occur:

- Remain calm and sympathetic. Lecture-free zones keep communication open.

- Avoid accusatory "why" questions. Say "this happened, now what can you do?"

- Discuss constructively how he could handle the situation better next time.

- Brainstorm together how to fix, or at least improve, the result.

- Note skills he applied effectively even amid the mishap.

With your steady guidance, he learns to reframe missteps as chance for growth.

Moving on After Disappointment

When a letdown occurs like a punishment, failed test, or not making a desired team, acknowledge the sadness. But also:

- Validate feelings of disappointment as normal.

- Put the setback in perspective - one event does not determine worth.

- Point out how coping well models maturity and strength.

- Note opportunities ahead to keep working towards goals.

- Suggest writing, talking to a friend, or exercise to process emotions.

- Do an activity he enjoys to lift spirits.

Supporting healthy coping prevents setbacks festering into lingering discouragement.

Owning and Apologizing for Mistakes

When your son misbehaves, guide sincerely apologizing by:

- Explaining clearly how the actions impacted others.

- Asking him to take responsibility for poor choices, not attribute to ADHD.

- Role playing a sincere apology and restorative plan.

- Having him apologize directly to those affected.

- Generating ideas to do better, then helping implement them.

- Expressing your unconditional love despite the mistake.

View missteps through a lens of empathy and accountability. Sincerity builds character.

Forgetting Perfection

Boys with ADHD often fixate on mistakes, viewing them as personal defects rather than opportunities to improve. Counter obsessive perfectionism by:

- Noting everyone makes mistakes - they are human.

- Praising effort over outcomes. Progress trumps perfection.

- Encouraging laughs at silly blunders to reduce shame.

- Reminding him that you love him just as he is.

- Celebrating qualities like creativity, enthusiasm, humor.

- Making lighthearted family "blooper reels" of slip-ups.

- Letting small failures happen without overreacting.

Lightening up around imperfections prevents hyper-self criticism.

Handling Emotional Fallout Compassionately

ADHD and emotional regulation challenges means meltdowns will occur when your child feels overwhelmed. During these moments:

- Remain the calm in the storm. Lower voices and model taking deep breaths.

- Give space while ensuring safety if emotions become explosive. Never punish outbursts.

- Listen sympathetically once emotions settle. Reflect his feelings back.

- Discuss what may have triggered the eruption and better ways to cope next time.

- Reassure your unconditional love and support.

With patience and nurturing guidance, he will gain skills to express upset feelings constructively over time.

Instilling Optimism and Resilience

Themost valuable mindset you can impart to your son is believing future success is always possible through perseverance. Teach resilience by:

- Noting how struggles often precede achievements.

- Reading stories of prominent people who overcame childhood ADHD.

- Saying "not yet" versus "I can't" when skills are under-developed.

- Considering setbacks temporary roadblocks rather than permanent barriers.

- Setting small goals to experience regular success.

- Encouraging positive self-talk about effort, not innate ability.

Your unwavering faith in him, despite obstacles, becomes his inner voice. Plant seeds of hope.

With abundant praise for milestones paired with calm optimism when facing setbacks, your son builds resilience to believe he can conquer any challenge. Celebrate every step while cultivating emotional tools to weather the valleys. Your steadfast guidance lights the path so he can take pride in the climb.

CONCLUSION

As the parent of a child with ADHD, you have been given the profound privilege of shepherding a wonderfully unique boy through the joys and struggles of growing up differently neurologically. The pages you've just read aim to provide practical knowledge and advice for fully supporting your son's needs with wisdom and compassion at each age and stage.

Yet while information is indispensable, what matters most on this journey cannot be encapsulated in a book. It is the profound, unconditional love you shower this child with every single day. It is the resilience you model in the face of hurdles. It is the laughter that carries you through difficult moments. And it is the deep, abiding faith you nurture in your son's inner strength, talents, and worthiness.

Parenting a child with ADHD is filled with peaks and valleys. There are dark days when you will feel utterly spent and at your rope's end over behavioral issues. And there are glowing days when your heart nearly bursts seeing your child's progress and delighting in his quirky personality. What remains constant is your essential role as his nurturer and champion.

You have the sacred task of teaching your son to believe in himself with unshakeable conviction. Though the outside world may try to label or limit him, your love drowns those voices out. Help him define himself not by a diagnosis but by his creativity, humor, empathy and passion. Show him that mistakes are opportunities, not indictments on self-worth. Install faith that he can conquer any challenge through perseverance. And remind him regularly that his unique wiring is a gift, not a flaw.

Take pride in parenting an extraordinary boy. The challenges of ADHD will evolve over time. But the incredible light within your child will only grow brighter. Whatever triumphs and trials may come, hold onto the following truths:

You've got this. No child could ask for a more devoted parent.

Your son is lucky to have your unconditional support.

With your guidance, he can achieve anything he dreams.

This is not a journey you walk alone - surround yourself with support.

There is no stronger advocacy than a mother's love. You are his superhero.

parenting child with ADHD will let you witness daily miracles.

The path may wind and bend but leads to a beautiful life. Have hope.

And above all else, trust your instincts. You know your son better than any expert. Listen to your heart, and you cannot go wrong. This child is yours to nurture, champion, and launch into a world that will be better for knowing him. What an honor it is to be his parent. Savor the extraordinary privilege.

BONUS

AUDIOBOOK

Scan The QR CODE

EXCLUSIVE BONUS

3 EBOOK

Scan the QR code or click the link and access the bonuses

http://subscribepage.io/4zgEy9

Made in the USA
Monee, IL
10 January 2024